PSYCHOPATHS

AN INTRODUCTION

Psychopaths
An Introduction
Herschel Prins

ISBN 978-1-904380-92-4 (Paperback)
ISBN 978-1-908162-32-8 (Adobe E-book)
ISBN 978-1-908162-33-5 (Kindle /Epub E-book)

Cover design © 2013 Waterside Press. Design by Verity Gibson/www.gibgob.com

Cataloguing-In-Publication Data A catalogue record for this book can be obtained from the British Library.

e-book *Psychopaths* is available as an ebook and also to subscribers of Myilibrary and Dawsonera.

Printed by MPG Books Group, Bodmin and King's Lynn.

Main UK distributor Gardners Books, 1 Whittle Drive, Eastbourne, East Sussex, BN23 6QH. Tel: +44 (0)1323 521777; sales@gardners.com; www.gardners.com

USA and Canada distributor Ingram Book Company, One Ingram Blvd, La Vergne, TN 37086, USA. (800) 937-8000, orders@ingrambook.com, ipage. ingrambook.com

Published 2013 by
Waterside Press Ltd.
Sherfield Gables
Sherfield on Loddon
Hook, Hampshire
United Kingdom RG27 0JG

Telephone +44(0)1256 882250
E-mail enquiries@watersidepress.co.uk
Online catalogue WatersidePress.co.uk

PSYCHOPATHS

AN INTRODUCTION

HERSCHEL PRINS

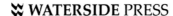 **WATERSIDE** PRESS

Dedicated to my post-graduate students in criminal justice and forensic mental health, past, present and future. With affection and respect.

Contents

Acknowledgements

My thanks are due to my friend and colleague, Dr Sarah Hodgkinson, for helpful discussion of a number of issues raised in the text.

Thanks to Joanne Forshaw of Routledge for permission to reproduced *Diagram 3(1)* and some subsequent text from *Chapter 3* of *Offenders, Deviants or Patients: Explanations in Clinical Criminology* (4th Edn., 2010).

To Mrs Janet Kirkwood for her continuing excellent word-processing skills and producing order out of chaos in my barely decipherable drafts.

Finally, thanks to Bryan Gibson, Director of Waterside Press for his editorial support and for compiling the *Glossary*. Also, his patience in waiting for the delivery of the manuscript, occasioned by a period of serious ill-health.

About the Author

Professor Herschel Prins began his 60-year involvement in the criminal justice and forensic mental health systems as a probation officer. This was followed by a period at the Home Office Probation Inspectorate and subsequent periods of university teaching, which continue at Leicester University. He has served on the Parole Board, the Mental Health Review Tribunal and the Mental Health Act Commission. He has also chaired three mental health inquiries and seen service on a number of committees concerned with crime and forensic mental health. His services to the latter have been recognised by having a low secure mental health unit at the Glenfield Hospital, Leicester named after him — The Herschel Prins Centre.

'I feel terrible about what happened all the more because I do not know why or what made me do it. I find it all a confusing matter. You see I'm scared of myself. At times I often try to wonder why, but it's just plain Hell'.

Statement by Patrick Mackay in Psychopath: The Case of Patrick Mackay by Tim Clark and John Pennycate (1975), London: Routledge.

'There's always a cause, no matter how terrible the crime, *always*. And I think we have to be willing to go into the darkness in order to achieve some kind of resolution'.

The psychiatrist, Sarah Trevelyan in an interview with Carol Ann Lee in her biography of Myra Hindley, One of Your Own: The Life and Death of Myra Hindley (2010), Edinburgh: Mainstream Publishing, p 378.

'I can't define an elephant, but I know one when I see one'.

Curran, D and Mallinson, P, 'Psychopathic Personality' (1944), Journal of Mental Science, 90: pp 266-280.

'What's in a name? That which we call a rose By any other name would smell as sweet'.

Juliet in Romeo and Juliet, Act 2, Scene 2.

They are 'Manfred-like characters, existing in their own time and space'.

Comment by the doyen child psychiatrist Dr Emmanuel Miller, in conversation with the author of this book in the late-1950s.

Preface: A Brief Historical Perspective

'Be afraid, be very afraid'.

From the feature film *The Fly*

Contemporary concerns and fears about madness and badness are fuelled by the media in their various guises. This can tend to give the less well informed the impression that such concerns and fears are of comparatively recent origin. Even a cursory inquiry into both history and literature demonstrates that this is not the case. It is also a truism that today we live in what has been aptly described as a 'risk society' (Beck, 1998) and a 'safety culture' (Tidmarsh, 1998; see also Prins, 2010).

Preoccupation with safety and danger — both real and imagined — has always been present. For example, in times of war the United Kingdom has invoked the Defence of the Realm Act 1914 (DORA) to provide for the detention of those considered to be a danger to the State; in other words those who are seen as 'aliens'. Similar provisions are invoked today, allowing for the detention of those thought to be a possible threat to the State through the planning and commission of terrorist acts. There are more subliminal examples; the fear of 'strangers' coming to our shores as immigrants, particularly if they are dark skinned. The use of the word 'alien' is apposite here with its connotation of 'difference', and described in Gothic literature as 'the other'.

In earlier periods of history the Common Law gave priority to the maintenance of law and order. However, exceptions could be made. For example, the Old Testament indicates that those who killed unintentionally could be ordered to be detained in one of the Cities of Refuge instead of being executed; this could be seen perhaps as an early example of punishment for the crime of manslaughter. However, against these examples of less Draconian measures it should be noted that during the Middle Ages the high security afforded by prisons had made them the most convenient places for the dangerously insane (for further discussion of this aspect see Walker and McCabe, 1973, p. 18).[1]

Such provision was not at all satisfactory and John Howard, the redoubtable explorer of penal treatment, in his classic study *The State of the Prisons* (1777) observed that:

> In some few gaols are confined idiots and lunatics. These serve for sport to idle visitants at assizes and other times of general resort. Many of the bridewells are crowded and offensive, because the rooms which were designed for prisoners are occupied by the insane. Where these are not kept separate they disturb and terrify other prisoners. No care is taken of them, although it is probable that by medicines, and proper regimen, some of them might be restored to their senses, and to usefulness in life.

---

1. For 'literary' depictions of those living and working during various periods within the Middle Ages, see for example Chaucer's *Canterbury Tales* and Langland's *Vision of Piers Plowman*. Clinical depictions may be found in Basil Clarke's detailed account of mental disorders in earlier Britain up to the Middle Ages. Clarke also explores the mental disorder suffered by Henry VI. For accounts of the early Vagrancy Acts, notably the Act of 1714, and for the discussion of the Poor Law Act of 1601, see Kathleen Jones (1993). See also Forshaw and Rollin (1990) who also cover the development of forensic psychiatry in England as well as a more recent contribution by Sugarman and Oakley (2012). For a short account of homelessness and vagrancy see Lodge-Patch (1990). The development of forensic psychiatry is also well illustrated in the series of biographies of pioneers in the field published in the *Journal of Forensic Psychiatry* over approximately a ten-year period. Arnold (2008) has published an insightful and detailed account of the role played by Bedlam (Bethlem Hospital) in the management and mismanagement of London's mad and bad. The fears engendered by the Black Death are described graphically in Hatcher's (2008) account of the disease in his study of one Suffolk village—Walsham. For a scholarly account of the relationship between the notion of a 'dangerous class' and various forms of sexual deviancy see Roudinesco (2009), particular her Chapter 3.

As I hope to demonstrate later in this book, the appropriate location of the so-called 'insane' in their various presentations (such as the psychopathic) has spawned numerous inquiries and legislative provision, but considerable problems remain. One of these concerns is the extent to which these might infringe the liberty of the subject. The dilemma was well described in a report by a Parliamentary Committee some four decades ago:

> Too much freedom for the patients would be dangerous to the public, but excessive restriction on the movement and association of patients would not only impede treatment but also increase the threat to security by providing boredom and tension among the patients. The public must be provided with strong protection against the most serious risks and with adequate protection against lesser risks ... But to make the security the overriding aim would, in our view, be incompatible with the therapeutic function of the hospitals.
>
> House of Commons Estimates Committee, 1968.
>
> Quoted in Walker and McCabe, 1973, p.14.

The problem of risk versus liberty in high security was addressed by Sir Richard Tilt, one time Director General of Her Majesty's Prison Service (HMPS). He and his colleagues came down heavily in favour of security as the overriding concern (Tilt *et al*, 2000; Tilt, 2003). Tilt and his colleagues seem to be somewhat 'at odds' with the members of the Estimates Committee some four decades earlier. For helpful discussion of the need to balance the rights of the individual and the need for public protection see two thought-provoking books by my one-time colleague Kate Moss (Moss, 2009; and Moss, 2011).

To return to earlier history and Elizabethan times, the eminent social historian Sir George Trevelyan depicted some of those who engendered fear among the populace. These were the 'sturdy beggars' who, by all accounts, were a motley crew. They consisted of

... the ordinary unemployed, the unemployable, soldiers discharged
after French wars and the Wars of the Roses ... serving men set
adrift by impecunious lords and gentry.

Trevelyan, 1946, pp 112-113.

Trevelyan adds that 'the cry "the beggars are coming" preyed
upon the fears of dwellers in lonely farms and hamlets and exer-
cised the minds of Magistrates, Privy Councillors and Parliaments'
(*Ibid*, p 113).

Such concerns can also be understood against fears prompted by
the Black Death. Although its pandemic proportions ravaged the
populace in the late-14th century, it continued to make its presence
felt well into Elizabethan times and later. The need to institute measures to control those who were different, and therefore dangerous,
found eventual expression in the Poor Law Act of 1601. This enact-
ment essentially legislated for the suppression of the mendicancy
(depending on alms or handouts for a living; begging) of 'rogues,
vagabonds and other disorderly persons'.

Today's older readers of this book may well recall seeing late
middle-aged and older itinerants carrying their few belongings on
their journeys from one reception centre to another (These had
been set up under the National Assistance Act of 1948). With the
closure of these centres in more modern times such itinerants seem
to have disappeared from view. Although in the main of harmless
intent, such people could at times cause alarm, largely because of
their sudden incomprehensible utterances. It has been suggested
that some of these sad folk were probably 'burnt-out' simple schiz-
ophrenics. Occasionally, their behaviour would bring them to the
attention of the emergency medical services or the police; and very
occasionally a court appearance if their behaviour constituted a
public order offence.

The Purpose of this Book

This book is not intended as a definitive text. Its aim is to present, in concise yet cogent form, an introduction and orientation to the vexed and vexing condition known as 'psychopathic disorder'. Such a disorder can, in some respects, be seen at the far end of a large spectrum of personality disorders in general. More recently, some see it as a separate condition.

I hope the book will be of value to undergraduates and post-graduates in criminology (particularly those taking an option in clinical criminology), psychology (particularly forensic psychology) and law. I trust it will also be of interest to a wide range of practitioners in the criminal justice system (for example, probation/offender management and prison staffs as well as the police, sentencers, both full-time and 'lay', and forensic mental health practitioners such as psychiatrists, psychologists and nurses, whether hospital or community-based). I hope also that it may have a more general appeal to interested members of the public.

In his introduction to Kurt Schneider's classic work *The Psychopathic Personalities* (first published in 1923), the late Professor Anderson, Professor of Psychiatry at Manchester University, alluded to the difficulties involved in attempting to define the term 'psychopathic' and how 'it had won for itself a mantle of opprobrium that attaches to hysteria'. Although our understanding of hysteria has now moved on since Anderson wrote those words, the same cannot be said with any degree of certainty about psychopathic disorder. I trust that the material conveyed in the following chapters will shed some light on a condition that has come to be described as the 'Achilles Heel' of psychiatry and psychology.

References, Further Reading and Food for Thought

Finally, I hope that readers will feel encouraged to consult more detailed or specialist works in order to expand the knowledge and information that is provided in the this modest account. With this in mind, I have not only provided a *Select Bibliography* but also some more targeted suggestions for further reading at the end of each chapter.

Similarly and with the intention of encouraging readers fresh to the subject in particular, I have added a number of questions at the end of chapters.

We have also added a *Glossary* of terms at the end of the book.

Chapter One
Origins and Orientation

'A mighty maze! But not without a plan'.

Alexander Pope, *An Essay on Man*, Epistle 1 (1733).

I need to emphasise that in this book we are dealing mainly with the *criminal* psychopath; that is someone who has shown psychopathic behaviour and become involved in the criminal justice and/or the forensic mental health care systems. There are others who demonstrate 'psychopathic' characteristics but who have not come to the notice of these systems. In an interesting article, Board and Fritzon described the extent to which some of those occupying senior management positions showed a number of characteristics seen in those who had been designated as criminally psychopathic (Board and Fritzon, 2005).

Pioneers — and a Little Social History

Those who have examined the historical development of the concept of psychopathic disorder have usually begun with the work of the early 19th century alienists (latter-day psychiatrists) Philippe Pinel, Jean Etienne Esquirol and the alienist/anthropologist James Cowles Prichard. The work of these three is illustrative of the burgeoning interest in criminal behaviour shown by medical practitioners. An example of this development may be found in the growing medical interest in fire-raising in the 19th century (see Prins, 1994, p 9). It is not entirely clear from an examination of the literature why this interest in forensic matters came about, but it seems reasonable to assume that it was an example of the 'scientific' approach to mentally disordered behaviour generally. McCord and McCord, in their book *Psychopathy and Delinquency,* make a sobering observation:

> Anyone who writes on the psychopathic personality faces a compli-
> cated, often puzzling task … [They] … must disentangle the various
> meanings of [this] ambiguous term … and then [they] must evaluate
> a mass of evidence concerning the nature, causes and treatment of
> the syndrome (1956: p ix).

Although, as stated above, most medically based accounts of the interest in psychopathic disorder usually begin with the work of the three aforementioned pioneers, history and literature reveal that its occurrence has a long history. In a series on history in the Old Testament, the psychiatrist George Stein (2009) asks whether 'the Scoundrel (Belial) in the Book of Proverbs was a psychopath?' And an American academic, Dr Eric Altschuler, of the University of California, suggests that, as a child, Samson may well have shown psychopathic characteristics, 'setting fire to things, torturing animals and bullying other children'.

Altschuler also refers to Samson's mother as a possible pathogenic element in his development. Apparently, in the Book of Judges 'she is warned not to drink when she is pregnant'. He concludes (perhaps somewhat with tongue in cheek) that 'recklessness and a disregard for others may have run in the family'. It is perhaps only fair to point out that the 'triad' of enuresis (which is *not* indicated in Alschuler's account) — with cruelty to animals and fire-setting, has in the past been noted as a precursor of later serious anti-social personality disorder.[1]

Those demonstrating what many would regard as psychopathic characteristics appear throughout post-Biblical times. For example, the nobleman Gilles de Rais (1404-1440) — a contemporary of Jean D'Arc — was a sadistic serial sexual killer of hundreds of children of both sexes. Vlad the Impaler (1441-1477; though dates vary) would probably be given the label of psychopath today.

---

1.   See *The Independent*, 15 February, 2002, which cites an unsourced paper in the *New Scientist*.

Literary Allusions

Tudor literature abounds with examples. Shakespeare provides numerous insights into characters showing psychopathic traits. For example, the general Titus Andronicus and his involvement in a series of bloodbaths of murder, cannibalism, rape and torture. Similarly, Iago, in his fervid jealousy of Othello's success and his depiction of Richard III (which, it must be stated, bears little relationship to that monarch's actual character).[2] Clues also of the possible genesis and manifestation of psychopathic disorder find insightful illustration in the scene in which Richard's aged mother, the Duchess of York, reviles him as follows:

> Thou cams't on earth to make the earth my Hell.
>
> A grievous burden was thy birth to me;
>
> Tetchy and wayward was thy infancy;
>
> Thy schooldays frightful, desp'rate, wild and furious;
>
> Thy age confirmed, proud, subtle, sly and bloody
>
> More mild, but yet more harmful, kind in hatred;
>
> What comfortable hour can'st thou name
>
> That ever grac'd me with thy company?

Shakespeare, *Richard III*, Act 4, Scene 4.

In this quotation we have the duchess describing graphically some of the features regarded by many people as being of possible importance in terms of aetiology (causes) and presentation. For example, an apparently difficult birth, longstanding anti-sociality which then becomes progressively more marked in adulthood. All of this accompanied by a veneer of charm and sophistication which serves to mask the underlying chaos and the potential for violent destructiveness. Some of these features will be addressed later in this book.

---

2. And the discovery of Richard III's skeleton in Leicester has provoked new interest in this respect.

Another of Shakespeare's characters, Lady Macbeth, provides us with a compelling illustration of serious personality disorder coupled with an eventual descent into severe depression—a case of dual diagnosis perhaps—not uncommon in the field of psychiatry (See Prins, 2001). In Chapter 40 of his classic book *The Mask of Sanity*, Hervey Cleckley (1976) provides numerous descriptions of individuals showing psychopathic characteristics, if not perhaps full-blown psychopathy as we might define it today. As examples he cites, Heathcliffe in *Wuthering Heights*, Iago in *Othello* 'perhaps the most interesting and ingenious creation of vindictiveness known to man' (p 353), and Dostoyevsky's Prince Myshkin in *The Idiot*.

Examples of developmental 'faults' in children may be found in Richard Hughes' *A High Wind in Jamaica*, and with frightening accuracy in Henry James' *The Turn of the Screw*. Contemporary examples may be seen in Brian Masters' account in *Gary* in his attempts to take into his home an adolescent psychopath (Masters, 1990), and in Lionel Shriver's compelling novel *We Need to Talk About Kevin* (Shriver, 2008). Her description of Kevin's mother's attitude to his conception, birth and development remind us in vivid fashion of an important element in child-mother relationships in the genesis of early anti-sociality, which may progress into serious and persistent criminality in adulthood.

In the past, much stress has been placed upon inadequate parenting and bonding. Responsibility for this has been laid frequently at the door of the parent (particularly the mother). But what if, for complex neuro-psycho-physiological reasons, the child is not able to respond to maternal cues and clues? This would certainly seem to be the case in Shriver's account of Kevin's history (above).

The vital question concerning maternal attachment and bonding is developed later in this book. Other depictions of the psychopathic character may be found in an early novel—James Hogg's *The Private Memoirs and Confessions of a Justified Sinner*, published in 1824. And, much more recently, in Sebastian Faulks' novel *Engleby* (2007).

Clinical Accounts

From these brief (and, it must be admitted, somewhat idiosyncratically selected) literary allusions, I now turn to more clinical accounts of psychopathic character and behaviour which have been described and discussed from the beginning of the 19th century to the present day.

As early as 1812, Benjamin Rush had drawn attention to the disorder:

> How far the persons whose diseases have been mentioned should be considered as responsible to human or divine laws for their actions, and where the line should be drawn that divides free agency from necessity and vice from disease, I am unable to determine.
>
> Quoted in McCord and McCord at p 22.

The problem, as stated by Rush, would still seem to be with us today. Consider, for example, the continuing debate concerning the defence of diminished responsibility in murder cases (see, for example, Hodgkinson and Prins (2011); Morris and Blom-Cooper (2011)). McCord and McCord point out that

> Throughout the 19th century investigation into the causes and treatment of psychopathy was buried in speculative dispute. Those who thought about the problem concerned themselves with theoretical [issues] like … can the moral sense be diseased and the intellectual faculty remain unimpaired?

However, the McCords also drew attention to the important fact that the 19th century witnessed the 'first faltering attempts' to study the *nature* of psychopathy. But, 'because of loose classification and lack of research, psychiatric pioneers accomplished little, yet they stimulated an intellectual movement which, by the early 1900s, had begun to build a store of observational data' (McCord and McCord, pp 22-23).

Reference has already been made to three 'pioneers' in this field, Philippe Pinel, Jean-Etienne Esquirol and James Cowles Prichard. What follows is a highly summarised account of their respective contributions. If their explanations are considered somewhat 'old-fashioned' by today's standards, readers should bear in mind that their work needs to be seen against a background of the rather primitive knowledge bases within both psychiatry and psychology at the time; it would be reasonable to describe both disciplines as nascent.

Phillipe Pinel

Pinel (1809) is usually cited as the first physician to describe so-called psychopathic disorder. However, by today's diagnostic standards, we would be far less certain that the condition he described as being representative of psychopathy in his three illustrative cases would satisfy today's criteria. The first is the frequently quoted case of the man who threw a woman into a well who, the man alleged, had been annoying him. The man in question had a history of cruelty to animals and engaged in severely impulsive behaviour. His second case showed periodic attacks of 'furor'. His third case showed marked agitation and aggression. According to Berrios, in his seminal analysis of the history of the concept of personality disorders, Pinel coined the descriptive term *manie sans délire*, a state of disordered affect, but without demonstrable illness as such (Berrios, 1993). His classification had its supporters and detractors. According to Berrios, Esquirol was 'unhappy with *manie sans délire*; he rarely, if ever, used the term' (Berrios, p 25). Esquirol raised the question, 'Can there be a pathological state in which men are irresistibly led to perform acts that their conscience rejects? I do not think so' (Esquirol, 1838, quoted in Berrios, p 25). The discerning reader will conclude that the debate continues to the present day.

James Cowles Prichard

These classificatory propositions were carried forward by Prichard, alienist and anthropologist, in his concept of 'moral insanity'. He described it as follows

> A madness, consisting of morbid perversion of the natural feelings, affections, inclinations, tempers, habits, moral dispositions and mental impulses, without any remarkable disorder of the intellect or knowing or reasoning faculties, and particularly *without any insane illusion or hallucination*.
>
> Prichard, 1835, p 26. Emphasis added.

Berrios considers that Prichard '[Did] ... for British Psychiatry what Pinel had done for his own: broke away from the intellectualist definition and widen[ed] the boundaries of insanity to the point that symptoms affecting other mental function might be significant to make a diagnosis' (p 27). As I shall note in a subsequent chapter, Prichard's views do find a degree of resonance in the work of Cleckley.

Other developments

Another 19th century development saw the creation of the term 'moral imbecility', possibly from the Lombrosian notion of the 'born criminal' (Lombroso, 1896/7; see also Feracutti, 1996).

Towards the end of the century Koch (1891) had formulated his concept of 'psychopathic inferiority', implying that the condition was caused by a constitutional pre-disposition. As McCord and McCord state 'In time, "constitutional psychopathy" gained wide use' (p 23). Koch's emphasis on constitutional factors was doubtless helped to prominence through the contemporary development of the importance of genetic and hereditary factors in behaviour pioneered in the United Kingdom by the work of Francis Galton and others.

These constitutional views (held by workers such as Charles

Mercier) seem to have found a place in England's Mental Deficiency
Act of 1913 where the proposed ingredients of psychopathy found
an outlet in such legal terminology as 'strong vicious and criminal
propensities' on which punishment seemed to have little effect.

At about this time, in the USA, Bernard Glueck, a prison psychiatrist, conducted a major study in Sing Sing Prison (Glueck,
1918). He 'found that the psychopaths had the greatest recidivism,
the highest proportion of drunkenness and drug addiction and the
earliest onset of anti-social behaviour' (McCord and McCord, p 23).
Glueck's summary of symptomatology, as quoted by the McCords,
seems to have been a precursor of much of the thinking on aetiology
(causation) that was to follow in the 20th century. Glueck's views
possibly helped to stimulate interest in what can best be described
as the study of developmental psychology and its relevance to persistent delinquency.

Sir Cyril Burt's classic study of juvenile delinquency in his book
The Young Delinquent (1944) endeavoured to chart the histories of
persistent youthful offenders. Burt's study arose out of his work as
an educational psychologist with the (then) London County Coun-
cil. His work is also notable for his employment of sophisticated
statistical techniques, a method that can be described as ground-
breaking for its time. Although his work in the field of education has
been the subject of considerable controversy concerning his alleged
manipulation of his statistics to support certain educational theories,
this alleged malpractice does not seem to have affected his work on
delinquency (See Prins, 1993). Burt's early exploration seems to have
provided a useful spur to long-term studies of delinquent careers,
notably the seminal work of Donald West and David Farrington.
West and Farrington conducted a series of studies of children from
the age of about seven and subsequently into adulthood. The work
of these two academics can be seen as of great importance for the
insights they have provided into the pathways producing later delinquency and criminality (West and Farrington, 1977; and West, 1982).

From the 1930s onwards interest in psychopathic disorder was

furthered by the work of those involved in psychoanalytic theoris-
ing and practice, early examples being studies by Franz Alexander,
Karpman and Lindner. The 1950s witnessed this earlier work
being continued by other psychoanalytically oriented medical and
non-medical professionals interested in the possible childhood
roots of later serious and persistent delinquency and criminality.
Exponents of this approach included, amongst others, Melitta
Schmideberg (daughter of Melanie Klein, the distinguished child
psychoanalyst), Kate Friedlander, Anna Freud (Sigmund Freud's
daughter) and those involved in running residential centres for
young persistent offenders such as August Aichorn in France and
George Lyward and Otto Shaw in the UK. The 'classical' psychoanalyst — Edward Glover — made a significant contribution in
suggesting that psychoanalytic insights could be relevant to the study
of serious criminality (see for example Cordess under *Suggestions for
Further Reading* at the end of this chapter).

In 1951 the editors of the (then) *British Journal of Delinquency*
(forerunner of the *British Journal of Criminology*) could suggest that:

> Psychopathy has now emerged as the most important of the great
> transitional [borderline] groups of mental disorders ... it occupies
> a fixed intermediate position in the hierarchy of developmental
> disorders ...

Editorial, British Journal of Delinquency, 2: 77. 1951.

It is of interest to note that the founding editors of this journal
illustrated an example of professional interest in juvenile delinquency and adult criminality. They were Edward Glover (already
mentioned), Emmanuel Miller (similarly) and Hermann Mannheim, the distinguished émigré criminologist at the London School
of Economics. In 1939, the British Professor of Psychiatry — Sir
David Henderson — published his well known work *Psychopathic
States* (1939). In it he divided psychopaths into three types — the
creative, the *inadequate* and the *aggressive*. Although his suggested

tripartite classification did not meet with universal acclaim, his work did suggest that a purely punitive approach to the last two of his categories would not be successful

> ' ... the psychopath's failure to adjust to ordinary social life is not a mere wilfulness or badness which can be threatened or thrashed out ... but constitutes a true illness'.
>
> Henderson, 1939, p 19.

His views are mirrored in the work of Cleckley. I return to these more 'therapeutic' views in my later discussion of management.

This period also saw other seminal studies within child psychology which focused attention on pathways to the development of serious anti-sociality. One early example of this work was the psychiatrist John Bowlby's study into the effect of maternal deprivation on the development of anti-social conduct. His first foray into the field was his classic study *Forty-four Juvenile Thieves* (Bowlby, 1946). An aspect of his important work has often been misquoted. He did not propose that the absence of the mother was *absolutely crucial*. What he *did* propose was that her place could be taken by an effective and maternal substitute.

Later contributions to the maternal care hypothesis were made by Ainsworth and others. For example, the film by the Robertsons — a husband and wife team — and accompanying book *A Two Year-Old Goes to Hospital* (Robertson films, 1952), demonstrated how harmful the absence of a mother at the child's bedside could be. In the days when the Robertsons made their film, parents were kept by hospital practice at a 'safe' distance. In the field of institutional care, Rene Spitz and others had demonstrated how lack of stimulation in child care institutions could produce 'frozen' children. Professor Lee Robins and, much later, Sir Michael Rutter have researched extensively into disturbances in childhood and their possible effect on later behaviour. Dr Bowlby continually revised and worked upon his early studies and formulated his important concept of 'attachment'. (More detailed information about all these workers may be found in Prins, 2010, Chapter 5).

Therapeutic Communities

Alongside these developments came the advent of the 'therapeutic community' approach to the management of severe anti-social personality disorder. A number of hospitals began to specialise in this area of forensic mental health work; examples being Dingleton Hospital in Scotland, the Cassell Hospital in London and the Henderson in Surrey.

Important figures at this time were the psychiatrists Maxwell Jones, Stuart Whiteley and, more recently, in Leicester, Penelope Campling. The therapeutic community approach in prison care had also been developing, and was pioneered at H M Prison Grendon Underwood (now known as Grendon). This type of institution within the penal system had been advocated in the pre-war report by Drs East and Hubert (Home Office, 1939). Its implementation had to wait until well after the Second World War. Such 'community' treatment had also been taking place within a small number of specialist units within the more conventional prison estate. In 2001, a second 'Grendon' opened at Dovegate Prison in Marchington, Staffordshire under private sector management. Later developments in the 'institutional' management of those showing serious anti-sociality have seen specialist units such as those at Whitemoor and Frankland Prisons and Rampton and Broadmoor high security hospitals for the treatment of those suffering from dangerous and severe personality disorder (below).

Dangerous and Severe Personality Disorder

It should be noted here that dangerous and severe personality disorder (DSPD) is a political 'invention' and not a clinical diagnosis (Home Office and Department of Health, 1999; and see *Chapter 3* for further discussion). The decision to establish such units was prompted by the lethal activities of Michael Stone, whose case is also discussed later and who had been well known to the mental health and criminal justice services (see Prins, 2007).

However, it is also probably true to say that there had been a more general political concern with psychiatry's *alleged* reluctance to deal with this particular group of individuals. There has been a considerable degree of controversy concerning the decision to establish specialist centres for the management of DSPD. In a well argued paper Tyrer *et al* suggest that the DSPD programme has not as yet proved its effectiveness and that its cost-effectiveness should be a matter of continuing scrutiny. However, the authors of this unbiased and clear review of the problem conclude that

> 'the DSPD programme *has helped to focus more general attention and resources on the treatment of those with personality disorder'* (emphasis added).

They state that 'England is the only country in the world that has a countrywide personality disorder service and none of this would have happened ... without the development of the DSPD programme' (Tyrer *et al*, 2010, p 96) (again, see also *Chapter 3*).

Neuro-physio-psychological and Other Approaches

In this brief history of the development of approaches to the diagnosis and management of psychopathic disorder limited reference has been made to neuro-physio-psychological approaches to the problem. Recent years have seen a considerable amount of research in this field and some of this is the subject of discussion in *Chapter 2*. However, readers wishing to orientate themselves at this stage will find the work of Blair and Frith (2000), Spence *et al* (2004), Blair *et al* (2005) and Patrick (2007) helpful.

Emerging Themes

It is difficult to summarise adequately the developments in thinking about psychopathic disorder as outlined here. A number of themes begin to emerge. The first, as Professor Coid (1993) has suggested, was the concept of abnormal personality as defined by social maladjustment, developed in France and subsequently in the United Kingdom. This led to the somewhat contentious legal definition of psychopathy in England and Wales, of which more in *Chapter 3*.

The second development was the concept of mental degeneracy—originally in France. Third, was the German notion of defining types of psychopathically disordered behaviours, as illustrated in the seminal work of Kurt Schneider (1958)(already mentioned in *Chapter 1*). In addition, over the years in the UK the concept has been addressed through the aegis of central government, for example in the report of the Butler Committee (Home Office and DHSS, 1975), the Reed Committee (Department of Health and Home Office, 1994), and in the Fallon Committee's report on its inquiry in the Personality Disorder Unit at Ashworth High Security Hospital (Fallon *et al*, notably Volume 2, 1999); and finally, as already mentioned, by the Home Office and Department of Health in their policy document concerning the measures needed for dealing with DSPD (Home Office and Department of Health, 1999).

In *Figure 1* I have attempted to further summarise these developments through the changes of nomenclature that have occurred from the beginning of the 19th century to the present day.

Figure 1: 'What's in a name?' From Pinel Esquirol and Prichard to the Home Office 1999

Mani sans deliré —> Moral insanity —> Moral imbecility —> (defectiveness) —> Mental Deficiency Act 1913 —> Constitutional psychopathic inferiority —> Neurotic character —> Psychopathy —> Sociopathy (USA) —> Anti-social personality disorder (Note 1) —> Dissocial personality disorder (Note 2) —> Dangerous and severe personality disorder (Note 3).

Notes

1. This term is in use in the *Diagnostic and Statistical Manual of Mental Disorders* (APA, 2005) and in the *International Classification of Mental and Behavioural Disorders* (World Health Organization, 1992).

2. *Ibid.*

3. The legal use of the term 'psychopathic' in England and Wales has, after much debate, now been deleted from statute. It is subsumed under the more general term 'mental disorder' in the Mental Health Act, 2007 (see further in *Chapter 3*).

4. Changes in *nomenclature* are often favoured in the hope that they may produce changes in *attitudes*. Professor John Gunn suggests that such changes may make a condition less 'horrid and worrying'. He adds that this notion can be exemplified 'in the history of the "privy", "the water closet", the "lavatory", the "toilet" or the "rest room"'. (Gunn, 2003, p 32). The value of a change of terminology may not always have the success that is desired. Many years ago the distinguished psychiatrist Eliot Slater espoused caution. He stated that 'if we were to drop the term ... [psychopathic disorder] ... altogether, we should be obliged to invent an equivalent or to overlook a wide range of clinically very important phenomena' (Slater, 1948).

Summary

I trust that a key consideration will have emerged from this introductory chapter, namely that psychopathic disorder can only be understood through a multi-disciplinary approach. The following vignette may help to illustrate this need. It appeared originally in an article written by the present author in the *Prison Service Jou*rnal in 1977 (Prins, 1977) (and in modified form in *Offenders, Deviants or Patients,* 4th ed, 2010, *Chapter 5*).

Vignette

Imagine, if you can, a top-level conference has been called to discuss the meaning of that much used and abused word *psychopathy*. You are privileged to be an observer at these discussions at which are present psychiatrists, psychologists sociologists, lawyers, sentencers, theologians, philosophers, staff of penal establishments and special hospitals, social workers and probation officers. You have high expectations that some total wisdom will emerge from this well-informed and experienced group of people and that a definition will emerge that will pass the closest scrutiny of all concerned. After all, this is a gathering of experts.

Alas, your expectations would have a quality of fantasy about them, for in reality you would find as many definitions as experts present. Let me just present one or two examples of this statement. There would be little agreement among psychiatrists; the term would be used to cover a very wide range of mental disorders, including those we in the UK might describe as neuroses; for some psychiatrists (for example, from the United States), the term might include minor disorders of personality and for others might be synonymous with what we would describe as recidivism.

The lawyers in the group would disagree also. Some might well accept the definition in the Mental Health Act 1959 (as it then was) which described psychopathy as a 'persistent disorder or disability of mind (whether or not including sub-normality of intelligence) which results in abnormally aggressive behaviour or seriously irresponsible conduct on the part of the patient and requires or is susceptible to medical treatment …'

However, they would immediately begin to ask questions about the legal implications of the words 'disability of mind' and 'irresponsible conduct'. At this stage, the philosophers would no doubt chip in and also ask searching questions about the same terms.

Later on in the discussion, a theologian might start asking awkward questions about the differences between 'sickness' and 'sin' and 'good' and 'evil'. The representatives from the field of sociology in the group might usefully remind us that psychopaths lack what they describe as a capacity for role-taking, i.e. seeing yourself in an appropriate role in relation to others in their roles in [their] environment. And so the discussion would go on and on.

Don't ever assume that it has been different. For 150 fifty years the arguments have raged over definition, classification and management.

Readers of this book could well ask, 'Have things changed much since that was written'? To which we would be forced to answer 'not much'. However, a group such as the one described in the vignette might well be somewhat more representative today. For instance, we could usefully find space for a geneticist, a developmental paediatrician, representatives from the Ministry of Justice and Department of Health, the voluntary sector (which does so much to cope with these 'hard to like' individuals) and perhaps, in this more progressive day and age, a consumer of the service as well as a victim?

Finally, Bavidge has suggested that

[Those] ... who wish to discuss issues of responsibility and the law [take on] ... the thankless task of stalking the boundaries between law, psychiatry and philosophy which, like most border territories, are matters of wars and disputes, of danger and confusion (Bavidge, 1989, p 11).

His statement forms a useful indicator of much that follows in the chapters to come.

Questions

1. Consider the following quotations:
   - 'History is more or less bunk' (Henry Ford, motor car magnate, 1916).
   - 'Those who cannot remember the past are condemned to repeat it' (George Santayana, *The Life of Reason*, 1905).[3]

   Having read this chapter, which of these quotations appeals to you most in relation to psychopathy and its related services?

2. Why is it important that everything is given a proper name?

---

3. I am grateful to Dr Conor Duggan OBE for bringing this quotation to my attention. Santayana's *The Life of Reason* is available in a 1998 edition in the series Great Books in Philosophy, Prometheus Books.

Suggestions for Further Reading

Between the years 1990-1996, the founding editor of the *Journal of Forensic Psychiatry* (Dr Paul Bowden) published a series of articles under the heading 'Pioneers in Forensic Psychiatry'.

Many of these articles throw light upon historical aspects of psychopathic disorder. A number of them are cited below, in order of their year of publication. All references are to that journal.

Bowden, P. (1990) 'Maurice Mamblin Smith'. 1: 103-113.

Bowden, P. (1991) 'William Norwood East: The Acceptable Face of Psychiatry'. 2: 59-78.

Cordess, C. (1992) 'Edward Glover' (1888-1972). Psychoanalysis and Crime – A Fragile Legacy'. 2: 509-530.

Bowden, P. (1992) 'James Cowles Prichard. Moral Insanity and the Myth of Psychopathic Disorder'. 3: 113-136.

Prins, H. (1993) 'Professor Sir Cyril Ludowic Burt: Delinquency and Controversy'. 4: 295-314.

Robertson, G. (1993) 'Professor T.C.N. Gibbens (1912-1983) Academic and Teacher'. 5: 551-568.

Bowden, P. (1994) 'Charles Arthur Mercier (1852-1919) Wit Without Understanding'. 5: 321-353.

Howard, C. (1995) 'Peter Duncan Scott (1914-1977). A Psychological Naturalist in the World of Deviance'. 6: 393-404.

Bowden, P. (1996) 'William Henry de Bargue Hubert (1904-1947) – Reformer and Expert Witness'. 7: 323-340.

Early historical development is covered in more detail in:

Maughs, S.B. (1941) 'A Concept of Psychopathy: Historical Development'. *Journal of Criminal Psychopathology* 2: 345-360.

Mallinson, P. (1944) 'Psychopathic Personality'. *Journal of Mental Science* 90: 266-280.

Gurvitz, M. (1951) 'Developments in the Concept of Psychopathic Disorder'. *British Journal of Delinquency* 2: 88-102.

The place of Henry Maudsley in the foregoing is well observed in Dr. Peter Scott's contribution in Hermann Mannheim's *Pioneers in Criminology*. (2nd edn.; Chapter 12). New Jersey: Patterson Smith.

Chapter Two
Mind Over Matter

'Myself when young did eagerly frequent
Doctor and Saint and heard great argument.
About it and about: but evermore came out
By the same door as in I went'.

The Rubáiyát of Omar Khâyyám, Stanza xxxvii[1].

'The wish to hurt, the momentary intoxication
with pain is the loophole through which the
pervert climbs into the minds of ordinary man'.

Jacob Bronowski, *The Face of Violence*,1954, Chapter 5.

Hopefully, readers who persist to the end of this chapter will be less despairing than the medieval Persian poet, mathematician and philosopher, Omar Khâyyám (1048-1131). And the quotation from the scientist Professor Jacob Bronowski provides a prefatory hint that in this book we are predominantly concerned with psychopathy's association with violence (most frequently a career of persistent violence). The so-called 'bad' Lord Byron hinted at the conflicting struggles within the mind of the psychopath, when he described 'the wandering outlaw of his own dark mind' (*Childe Harold's Pilgrimage*, Canto 3, Stanza 3, 1812-1848).

The material which follows is intended mainly as a guide to the manner in which brain function (or, more particularly, malfunction) may contribute to serious anti-social behaviour. Those wishing to take their studies further concerning this aspect should consult the *Select Bibliography* and *Suggestions for Further Reading*.

---

1.   Translated by Edward Fitzgerald, Oxford World Classics, Karlin, D (Ed.), 2010, Oxford: Oxford University Press.

Put simply (perhaps over-simply), the brain provides the thinking processes behind our behaviour and the heart provides the 'engine' which helps to produce it. To the layman and woman the brain tends to be conceived of as a single entity consisting of those 'little grey cells' beloved of Agatha Christie's Belgian detective Hercule Poirot. The content of the brain can be seen as a 'blancmange-like' mass surrounded by a tough skeletal structure which is difficult to penetrate. Sometimes, small babies may be shaken with the result that this developing floppy mass gets banged against the hard bony structure, occasionally with traumatic results.

A further way in which to envisage the brain is to see it not as a single working entity but as a structure containing a number of 'mini brains', each having particular functions. These mini-brains can all operate at the same time in order to deal with responses provoked by external sources. Some further confirmation of this statement may be found in a description of research carried out at a number of universities in the UK, USA, Geneva, Canada, Italy and more recently in the ground-breaking work of Baron-Cohen and his Cambridge colleagues (2011). This work I regard as seminal in this field. Research indicates, for example, that at least 12 different areas of the brain are involved in producing various emotional states. These findings have come about largely through the introduction of functional magnetic resonance imaging (fMRI). Researchers have also identified a large range of brain chemicals that in addition are involved in the process. The 'mini-brains' of greatest interest to those who study psychopathic behaviour (neuro-scientists in different disciplines, as to which see later in this chapter) are, to over-simplify somewhat, the pre-frontal cortex, the amygdala, and the hypothalamus.

Sir Arthur Conan Doyle's fictional detective, Sherlock Holmes, offers a vastly simplified account of some aspects of normal brain function:

'A Man should keep his little brain attic stored with all the furniture
he is likely to use, and the rest can be put away in the little room of
his library where he can get at it if he wants it'.

The Adventures of Sherlock Holmes: The Five Orange Pips,1892.

This statement is vastly oversimplified because it does not take
into account the many 'insults'—both psychological and physical—that may assail the brain in various ways. Many years ago
Mark and Irvin, in describing the brain as the organ of behaviour,
suggested that its organization and functions were dependent upon
four elements:

(1)   The physical structure of the brain and its chemical envi-
       ronment.
(2)   The moment to moment information being received by the
       brain from the outside world and the rest of the body [via
       the central nervous system].
(3)   The information stored in the brain from past experience.
(4)   The associations made in the brain between present and
       past information.

Mark and Irvin, 1970, p.6.

There is a common misapprehension that we only use ten per cent
of our brains at any one time. This is not quite correct. Different
parts of the brain have different functions, but these functions are
not entirely discrete and they may operate in conjunction with each
other. It is probably more correct to suggest that, overall, the various
functions of the brain are only partially understood. A neurologist
once informed me that the volume of this knowledge probably
stands at ten per cent or less, a sobering thought.

However, as I have suggested, advances in the neuro-sciences
have enabled us to understand much more than we did. As already
noted, they have come about largely as a result of the development
of sophisticated neuro-imaging techniques through the increasing

availability of scanning devices based upon MRI. As we learn more about which neurological 'faults' may affect behaviour (particularly seriously violent behaviour in particular) further questions are bound to arise. For example, to what extent should diagnosable 'faults' of this kind have a bearing upon the determination of criminal responsibility? A further area of much interest concerns the vexed question of the relationship between genetic factors and the social and close environmental life of an individual and their neurological implications. In other words, how does their interplay have implications for normal and abnormal development? This complex relationship has been the subject of a good deal of investigation and speculation in modern times giving rise to a whole new area of study—epigenetics. Readers are referred to Rutter (2006), Callender (2010) and Baron-Cohen (2011) for extensive discussion of these aspects. Callender expresses a clear need for continued studies in this field as follows:

> [The] task now is to understand the many ways in which gene expression and brain functioning are affected by a wide range of adverse environmental exposures. These include abuse, neglect, malnutrition, infection and doubtless many others whose significance is, as yet, unknown.
>
> Callender, 2010, p.134.

A Selection of Hazards

There are a number of hazardous occurrences that may impact upon brain function, and bring about serious personality change, which, in turn, *may* lead to serious anti-social (psychopathic) behaviour. I must emphasise that I am offering a selective account (indeed, some may consider my choices idiosyncratic). A number of them may have greater impact than others. Moreover, their importance may occasionally be overlooked. I have decided to use the term 'organic' since this word can embrace a variety of conditions (For a more comprehensive account of all these aspects see Prins, 2010, Chapter 4).

(1) Infections

Certain infective conditions (such as meningitis and encephalitis in childhood) may not only cause learning disability but, in addition, may produce behavioural disorders involving aggressive outbursts. It is perhaps worth noting here that a urinary tract infection in the elderly may sometimes be misdiagnosed as a stroke. Patients so suffering may become confused and aggressive. Treatment with antibiotics will usually bring about fairly speedy improvement.

(2) Huntington's disorder (formerly known as Huntington's chorea)

This is a directly inherited disorder. Its onset usually occurs in or around the forties. The eventual outcome is terminal. The general physical and mental deterioration of the sufferer may very occasionally be accompanied by aggressive outbursts.

(3) General paralysis of the Insane (GPI) — Neurosyphilis

This disorder occurs as a result of a primary syphilitic infection. It is far less common today because of earlier diagnosis and the availability of antibiotics. Serious behavioural changes may occur. The disordered behaviour may sometimes be misdiagnosed as an episode of hypo-mania unless a careful history is taken and neurological tests are carried out.

(4) Toxic substances

A history of chronic alcohol abuse may produce serious behavioural problems; its continued abuse may produce brain damage. For those individuals already exhibiting signs of such damage, the continued abuse of alcohol *even in very small amounts* may result in unprovoked episodes of serious violence. Alcohol and its relationship to serious sexual offending has been well documented. Its use is depicted in graphic form by the Porter in *Macbeth*. When asked by Macduff 'What three things does drink especially provoke?', the Porter replies (in relation to lechery):

'Lechery, sir, it provokes and unprovokes; it provokes the desire, but it takes away the performance. Therefore much drink may be said to be an equivocator with lechery: it makes him, and it mars him; it sets him on, and it takes him off; it persuades him and disheartens him, makes him stand to and not stand to'.

Macbeth, Act III, Scene 3.

Here we have in the most vivid terms the role of alcohol in relation to erectile function and performance. Drink is sometimes consumed in the hope that it will enhance sexual performance whereas, in fact, as alcohol is a cerebral depressant, it has the reverse effect.

The continued abuse of other drugs (for example cannabis, heroin, amphetamines, etc.) is likely in all these instances to produce episodes of serious anti-social behaviour. Less well known are the effects of certain chemicals (such as carbon tetrachloride, used in the dry-cleaning process) in producing serious behavioural changes. Although such instances may be rare, it is important to be aware of their possibility. In medieval and post-medieval times contaminated foodstuffs, such as ergot of rye in flour, produced major behavioural changes, often described as the 'dancing mania' because of the jerky choreiform movements it produced (see Camporesi, 1989). Other chemical substances have had their place, mercury being a good example. It was thought for a long time that Newton suffered from depressive episodes. Research, including analysis of his work, has shown subsequently that these episodes were most likely to have been caused by his inhalation of mercuric fumes in the course of his many experiments.

And Lewis Carroll gives us a hint that the so-called Mad Hatter in *Alice's Adventures in Wonderland* suffered from the same substance, since mercuric compounds were used in the making of felt hats (see Klawans, 1990). Arsenic (and its derivatives) had its place. In Victorian times it was used (and we could say abused) in the manufacture of various foodstuffs (such as confectionery) and in the decoration of houses and other buildings. All these instances could produce behavioural changes (see Whorton, 2010 for a fascinating history concerning many forms; and also Wilson, 2013).

(5) Metabolic and associated influences

Metabolic changes may influence behaviour to a significant degree (for example during pregnancy, the menstrual cycle and menopause). Associated states such as over-active thyroid function and untreated diabetes can also produce significant and serious behavioural changes (see Prins, 2010, Chapter 4 for details).

(6) Direct injury to the brain

In infancy and childhood

Direct assault on the brain of a developing child may result in serious changes in behaviour. Even minor assaults already referred to, such as shaking an infant, may result in long-term adverse effects which may not have registered with those caring for the child at the time. The latter may result in a degree of non-responsiveness on the part of the child, he or she merely noted as being 'difficult'. The parents (particularly the mother) may be blamed for a lack of parenting skills and a vicious circle is thus established. In other instances, the parent (frequently the mother) may be missing or, if present, be unable to demonstrate unconditional affection. It was in such instances that Dr John Bowlby developed his concept of the so-called 'affectionless character' (Bowlby, 1946).[2]

Despite the early misunderstandings of Bowlby's original proposition, and the problems inherent in understanding the complex

---

2.   Bowlby followed up his earlier work in this field in his book *The Making and Breaking of Affectional Bonds* (1979). The broader issues of maternal deprivation are described and discussed by Ainsworth in her report for the World Health Organization (1962). As already stated, further aspects of the effects of maternal deprivation were brought to attention vividly in the films made by James and Joyce Robertson between 1967-1972.

inter-relations between genetic and environmental factors, it is important to observe the extent to which severe emotional deprivation appears to be evident in the backgrounds of many of those who go on to exhibit serious anti-social conduct (psychopathy). Some of these complexities are illustrated poignantly in Lionel Shriver's novel (See *Chapter 1* of this volume).

In adulthood

An injury to the brain (brain trauma), however caused, may bring about behavioural changes, particularly if a degree of concussion was involved. Such changes are in marked contrast to the previous personality of the person so afflicted. A striking forensic example of such a change is that provided by the case of James Hadfield, who tried to assassinate King George III. Hadfield was tried for capital treason in 1800 for shooting at the king in the Theatre Royal at Drury Lane, London. Thomas Erskine, Hadfield's counsel, obtained his acquittal on the basis of Hadfield having sustained serious head injuries (through sword wounds) during war service. These injuries had led Hadfield to develop delusional ideas that impelled him to believe that he had to sacrifice his life for the salvation of the world. Not wishing to be guilty of suicide and the condemnation and obloquy this would call down upon his memory, he chose to commit his crime for the sole purpose of being executed for it. Readers wishing to seek more information concerning Hadfield's case, and the legal and administrative consequences that flowed from it, may care to consult Prins, 2010, p 23 *et seq*.

A well known non-forensic case is that of Phineas Gage. As a result of an explosives accident in 1848, whilst employed as a foreman on a railway, Gage sustained a wound from a rod that penetrated his face and forehead. This damaged his pre-frontal cortex. From being a 'well respected and organized individual ... [he became] ... a man who was garrulous, sexually promiscuous, reckless, unreliable and irresponsible—essentially a pseudo-psychopathic individual' (Damasio, 1994). In Hadfield's case his injury produced a severe mental illness (a psychotic delusional state), and in Gage's case a complete change of personality. Both suffered similar types of injuries, but presented with very different signs and symptoms. Those pertaining to Gage's case are probably of greatest relevance to our concern with psychopathy. For further discussion of this phenomenon see Raine and Yang (2007).

(7) Dementia and other disorders

There are various forms of dementia; the most quoted of these is Alzheimer's. Dementing processes are of limited importance in relation to psychopathic disorders. However, from time to time, cases occur where the possibility of a dementing process has not been recognised at an early stage. Any individual appearing in court, of hitherto unblemished record, who, out of the blue, commits a series of apparently inexplicable offences such as indecent assault or exposure, should be examined for the presence of possible psychiatric and, more particularly, neurological disorder.

Mention must also be made here of the possible role played by the presence of a tumour, be it malignant or benign. The primary site may be in the brain, or it may be a 'secondary' with the primary site elsewhere. My earlier remarks concerning the need for psychiatric and/or neurological examination apply with equal force here.

(8) Epileptic type disorders

Epilepsy (or rather the epilepsies in their various presentations), is (are) not generally significantly associated with persistent criminality. However, important research carried out some years ago by Professor John Gunn did find a raised incidence of epilepsy in a male prison population (Gunn, 1977) (For further discussion see Prins, 2010, Chapter 4).

One somewhat singular condition, considered to be of epileptic origin, has been described as 'episodic dyscontrol syndrome', 'limbic rage' or 'intermittent explosive disorder'. Opinions vary concerning the validity of the disorder and its designation as a form of pseudo-epilepsy (For a summary of some of the arguments for and against, see Prins, 2010, pp 140-141).

(9) Mental impairment (Learning disability).

There is no strong link between learning disability and persistent serious offending involving violence. However, I was involved some years ago in a case that demonstrates the possibility.

Vignette

A man of 26 was charged with causing grievous bodily harm to a young woman by hitting her over the head with an iron bar. She was entirely unknown to him, and though he denied the offence vehemently, he was convicted by (what is now) the Crown Court on the clearest possible evidence.

As a child he had suffered brain damage, which had resulted in a mild degree of mental impairment, accompanied by impulsive, aggressive and unpredictable behaviour. He had been before the courts on a number of occasions and had eventually been sent to a hospital for the mentally handicapped. He was discharged some years later to the care of his mother. Subsequent to his discharge, he committed the offence described above and was placed on probation. His response was poor. He was impulsive and erratic, and regressed to very childish behaviour when under stress.

The family background was problematic. The parents had divorced (acrimoniously) when the offender was quite small. A brother suffered from a disabling form of epilepsy and two other siblings showed decidedly eccentric lifestyles (No doubt today, such a family would be described as 'dysfunctional'). Shortly after the probation period expired, he committed a particularly vicious and unpro- voked assault on a small girl and was sentenced to a long term of imprisonment. Such a case reminds us of the complex inter-play of possible genetic and social/environmental factors.

What Is Personality?

Before moving on to consider neuro-scientific aspects in more detail, it seems appropriate to attempt to define what we mean when we discuss personality and, in particular, serious personality disorder. There have always been problems in defining personality with any degree of consensus. It is a word used in common parlance to cover a wide range of attributes and behaviours. An early and useful short definition was provided many years ago by Gordon Allport. He suggested that:

> 'Personality is the dynamic organization within the individual of those psycho-physical systems that determine his unique adjustment to the environment'.
>
> Allport, 1937, p.48 .

Trethowan and Sims (1983) have offered a slightly more detailed description:

> 'Personality may be either considered subjectively i.e. in terms of what the [person] believes and describes himself as an individual, or, objectively in terms of what an observer notices about his more consistent patterns of behaviour ... Personality will include such things as mood state, attitudes and opinions and all these must be measured against how people comport themselves in their social environments. If we describe a person as having a "normal" personality, we use the word in a statistical sense indicating that various personality traits are present in a broadly normal extent neither to gross excess nor extreme deficiency. Abnormal personality is, therefore, a variation upon an accepted yet broadly conceived range of personality' (p.9).

The words of a non-psychiatric professional offer a slightly broader 'take' on their definition. Miri Rubin—a medieval historian—writes:

> Personal and group identity is best thought of as a cluster of attributes and associations including aspects of age, gender, region, occupation, experience and training. *Areas of identity are always heightened when they seem most different.*
>
> Rubin, 2005, p 8 (Emphasis added).

When we consider what Trethowan and Simms (1983) describe as the *extremes* of personality, the two definitions of personality disorder as given in the *Diagnostic and Statistical Manual of Mental Disorders* (DSMIV) (APA, 2005) and *International Classification of Mental and Behavioural Disorders* (ICD 10) (WHO, 1992) amplify these. The DSMIV defines them as:

> 'An enduring pattern of inner experience and behaviour that deviates markedly from the expectations of the individual's culture, is pervasive and inflexible, has an onset in adolescence or early childhood, is stable over time, and leads to distress or impairment'.
>
> As quoted in NIMHE for England, 2003: 9.

The ICD 10 defines personality disorder in the following terms:

> 'A severe disturbance in the characterlogical and behavioural tendencies in the individual involving several areas of the personality, and nearly always associated with considerable personal and social disruption'.
>
> *Op. cit.*

As to *psychopathic* disorder more specifically, the DSM IV defines it in the following terms:

(A)   A pervasive pattern of disregard for, and violation of, the rights
        of others occurring since age 15 years as indicated by three (or
        more) of the following:

   (1)   Failure to conform to social norms with respect to lawful
         behaviour as indicated by repeatedly performing acts that
         are grounds for arrest.

   (2)   Deceitfulness, as indicated by repeated lying, use of aliases,
         or conning others for personal profit or pleasure.

   (3)   Impulsivity or failure to plan ahead.

   (4)   Irritability or aggressiveness as indicated by repeated physi-
         cal fights or assaults.

   (5)   Reckless disregard for safety of self or others.

   (6)   Consistent irresponsibility, as indicated by repeated failure
         to sustain consistent work behaviour or honour financial
         obligations.

   (7)   Lack of remorse, as indicated by being indifferent to
         or rationalising having hurt, mistreated, or stolen from
         another.

Three further criteria are listed in Section (B) of the definition

   (a)   The individual is at least age 18 years.

   (b)   There is evidence of conduct disorder before age 15 years.

   (c)   The occurrence of anti-social behaviour is not exclusively
         during the course of schizophrenia or a manic episode.

APA, 1994, pp 649-650.

As Lykken points out, the criteria adopted in the DSM 'could
include a number of heterogeneous individuals who we call common
criminals... as well as many feckless citizens who do not commit
serious crimes' (Lykken, p.4). The same criticism could be levelled
at the 16 criteria listed by Cleckley in his book *The Mask of Sanity*
(1976) which has already been mentioned in *Chapter 1*.

In similar fashion, Hare, in his book *Without Conscience*, alludes to the fairly ubiquitous nature of behaviours that may not fit the strict criteria of criminality. Hare suggested that such 'psychopathic' individuals may be found 'in business, the home, the professions, the military, the arts, the entertainment industry, the news media, and the blue collar world' (Hare, 1993, p 57).

It is no small wonder then that acceptable definitions and categorisations have been highly elusive. Lykken suggests that our fascination with the contradictions inherent in the make-up of the so-called psychopath, is illustrated in the case of Oskar Schindler, 'the saviour of hundreds of Krakov Jews'. He is described by Lykken as an 'opportunist, bon vivant, lady's man, manipulator, unsuccessful in legitimate business by his own admission, but wildly successful in the moral chaos of wartime'. Lykken suggests that

> 'Schindler's rescue of those Jews can best be understood as a 35-year-old conman's response to a kind of ultimate challenge. Schindler against the Third Reich' (p. 12).

Perhaps this characteristic can best be likened to the psychopath's need for a 'high' as suggested later in this chapter.

The World Health Organization subsumes psychopathic disorder under the heading of dissocial personality disorder (DPD) in the following fashion:

> Personality disorder coming to attention because of a gross disparity between behaviour and the prevailing social norms, and characterised by:
>
> (a) callous unconcern for the feelings of others;
> (b) gross and persistent attitude of irresponsibility and disregard for social norms, rules and obligations;
> (c) incapacity to maintain enduring relationships, though having no difficulty in establishing them;

(d)   very low tolerance to frustration and a low threshold for
       discharge of aggression, including violence;

(e)   incapacity to experience guilt or to profit from experience,
       particularly punishment;

(f)   marked proneness to blame others, or to offer plausible
       rationalisations for the behaviour that has brought the
       patient into conflict with society.

There may also be persistent irritability as an associated feature.
Conduct disorder during childhood and adolescence, though not
invariably present, may further support the diagnosis.

WHO, 1992, p.204.

It will be seen that the two classifications do not differ to any
marked degree. In my view, the WHO classification is more succinct
and perhaps more in line with UK thinking and practice.

Revisions of the DSM IV and the ICD10 are expected in the
near future. There is speculation that the new versions (notably
of the DSM IV) may add a number of 'problems of living' to the
existing manifold classifications (For an interesting commentary
on what the final outcome of such revisions might be,[3] see Kendler
and First, 2010).

In the UK, the term 'psychopathic disorder' (which many have
considered to be pejorative and confusing) has disappeared from
current legislation and is subsumed under the broad definition of
any disorder or disability of the mind (See Fennell, 2007, Chapter
3) and my comments in later parts of this book.

In summary, we may consider that the modern concept of personality disorder and, by implication, psychopathic disorder seems to
represent two interlocking notions. The *first* suggests that it is present
when any abnormality of personality causes problems, either to the
person themselves or to others. The *second* carries a more pejorative

---

3.   This outcome may be known in the course of 2013.

connotation; it implies unacceptable, anti-social behaviour incurring dislike for the person showing such behaviour and a rejection of them (see later). It is in embracing this latter interpretation that the term 'psychopath' is often applied.

Is it All in the Mind?

Introductory Comments

As already noted, interest has been revived concerning possible 'organic' causes, including both major and minor cerebral 'insults' in infancy and the consequences of obstetric complications. If such developments subsequently prove to have unequivocally firm foundations, one could envisage a situation where issues of responsibility (and notably diminished responsibility) may well have to be addressed by the courts. This is an arena already fraught with problems concerning the relationship between medicine (particularly psychiatry and neuro-psychiatry) and the law (see Spence *et al,* 2004; and Morris and Blom-Cooper, 2011 for useful discussions of this aspect). It has been suggested that the environment also plays a significant part in the aetiology (causes) of the disorder.

It may well be that, as with other mentally disturbed states such as the schizophrenias, it is the interplay of social forces and pressures acting upon an already vulnerable personality (arising for whatever reason) that may tend to produce the conditions. Again, as I have already suggested, some of the highly complicated and sophisticated neuro-physio-chemical research undertaken fosters speculation that *some* of the answers to the problem of aetiology may well be found in the area of brain structure and biochemistry.

Similar possibilities are of equal interest. For example, one cannot ignore the evidence, admittedly laboratory-based, of such factors as low anxiety thresholds, cortical immaturity (childlike patterns of brainwaves in adults), frontal lobe damage and, perhaps most relevant of all, the *true*, as distinct from the wrongly labelled, psychopath's need for excitement—the achievement of a 'high'. Such a need is described graphically in Wambaugh's (1989) account of the case of Colin Pitchfork.

Vignette

Colin Pitchfork was convicted of the rape and murder of two teen-age girls in Leicestershire during the period 1983-86. In interviews with the police, it is alleged he stated that he obtained a 'high' when he exposed himself to women (he had previous convictions for indecent exposure prior to his two major offences). He also obtained a 'high' from the knowledge that his victims or likely victims were *virgo intacta*. He is said to have described an additional aspect of his excitement, namely obtaining sex outside marriage. As with others assessed as psychopathic, he also demonstrated a great degree of charm; for example, he was able to get his wife to forgive him for a number of instances of admitted unfaithfulness (Pitchfork's case is also of interest in that it involved the earliest attempt to use DNA-profiling, a procedure pioneered by Professor Sir Alec Jeffreys at Leicester University. The procedure has become almost routine today).

Biochemical-neurophysiologic Approach and the Limbic System

It has been suggested that severe personality disorder (SPD) (i.e. psychopathic) might be caused by alterations of, or abnormalities in, the normal chemical processes of the brain, which in turn may adversely affect the motivational processes that guide thoughts and perceptions. Such alterations of the normal chemical processes of the brain, or brain activity, can result from brain diseases such as cancer, nutritional deficiencies, brain injury, pollutants (such as lead) and even hypoglycaemia (see earlier discussion).

In many instances such brain damage goes unnoticed, since the brain has an innate capacity to compensate itself for damaged areas. This appears not to be the case, however, where the limbic system is concerned. The limbic system is located in the upper brain stem and lower cerebrum portion of the brain. It is thought to be directly involved with brain processes relating to motivation and aggression. When the limbic system is damaged it can result in a person presenting with uncontrollable rage and violence. Such damage can be organic (as with the viral infection rabies, that specifically attacks the limbic system) or alternatively, as I have suggested, non-organic resulting from brain injury or trauma.

Such an approach is relatively new and unique, since it moots the possibility that a person's behaviour can be explained without necessarily having to refer to provocation by an external event.

The cerebral cortex

To date there has been *relatively* little systematic study of psychopathy from a neurological perspective. This is probably due to two reasons.

- *Firstly*, since, as already mentioned, psychopathy as a term is controversial and difficult to define, it follows that empirical research regarding such a broad and ill-defined term is difficult to carry out.

- *Secondly*, studying the neurobiology of cohorts of psychopaths is difficult because a great many psychopaths will never find themselves in a clinical psychiatric setting.

However, since the seminal work of Harvey Cleckley (1976), built upon by Robert Hare *et al* (1990) in their development of a research scale—the Psychopathy Checklist, now known as the Psychopathy Checklist-Revised (PCL-R) (see further in the *Glossary*)—it has been shown that valid and reliable research can indeed be carried out to predict recidivism in criminal populations. This is done using a two-factor structure, consisting first of personality traits such as glibness, lack of remorse and failure to accept responsibility, and second, anti-social traits and aggression. In this context the possibility of developing a neurobiological approach to psychopathy has become feasible.

Neurobiological underpinnings to this condition have been furthered in the findings of studies of the cerebral cortex using the electro-encephalogram (EEG). These have tended to show that the 'slow wave' activity of the brain of some aggressive psychopaths bears some degree of resemblance to the EEG tracings found in children. Such findings have led to the formulation of a hypothesis of cortical immaturity, which may explain why the aggressive behaviour of some psychopaths seems to become less violent with advancing years because, as in children, the brain matures.

Heredity

It is by now fairly well established that some types of personality disordered behaviour seems to run in families. Notwithstanding this, the nature versus nurture debate has continued. However, as McGuffin and Tharpar (2003) report:

> The evidence pointing to a genetic contribution to anti-social personality comes from three main sources (p 215).

These are:

- *Firstly*, studies on animals which point to a genetic component to some temperamental features such as aggression;

- *Secondly*, genetic research in relation to twins which has suggested that certain traits (including anti-social ones) are hereditary; and

- *Thirdly*, studies of criminality within families which indicate an hereditary component to both juvenile delinquency and adult anti-social conduct (see later discussion).

More recently, the study of molecular genetics is furthering understanding of the biological bases of inherited personality traits. One of the difficulties regarding the application of genetics to this area of study is that it remains uncertain as to whether psychopathy is a 'discrete entity', or whether it is a continuum of behaviour ranging from the blatantly pathological to the normal (see for example work by Roberts and Coid, 2007). I would suggest that the latter is more likely, but given the difficulty of defining this condition, the application of research in relation to it remains uncertain and problematic (see Waldman and Rhee, 2007). The study of molecular genetics may provide more certainty in the future.

Cortical under arousal

Research in the field of the neurosciences has also suggested that psychopathy may be linked with a defect or malfunction of certain brain mechanisms concerned with emotional activity and the regulation of behaviour. More specifically, cortical arousal refers to the situation where the brain is wide awake, attentive to stimulation and working at its maximum. Conversely, low cortical arousal refers to a lack of attention, tiredness and lack of interest. It has been suggested that psychopathy may be related to a lowered state of cortical excitability and to the attenuation of sensory input, particularly input that would, in ordinary circumstances, have disturbing consequences. This may partially explain the apparent callous and cold indifference to the pain and suffering of others which is demonstrated by some seriously psychopathically disordered individuals. This may also go some way to explain why certain psychopaths (particularly the seriously aggressive) may seek stimulation with arousing or exciting qualities and have reported that they derive a 'high' from their actions (see the earlier *Vignette* concerning the case of Colin Pitchfork).

As long ago as 1982, McCord stated that 'most psychopaths do not see security as a goal in itself; rather they crave constant change, whirlwind variety and new stimuli' (1982, p 28). Further, he suggested that Ian Brady and the late Myra Hindley illustrated the psychopath's craving for excitement, since the ways in which they behaved were 'simply ways to attain new levels of excitement, a new "consciousness" and a temporary escape from boredom'. This craving may render the psychopath unaware of many of the more subtle cues required for the maintenance of socially acceptable behaviour and for adequate socialisation—described by the present writer as a 'failure to register' (see Prins, 2010, Chapter 5; and in particular Baron-Cohen, 2011).[4]

Inability to learn/inconsequentiality

It has been postulated, since human behaviour is flexible and not fixed, that both criminal and non-criminal behaviours stem from the same general social-psychological processes and that, as such, many types of behaviour are learned, specifically through association with others. In the case of psychopathy however, it has been tentatively suggested that these individuals do not possess the same ability to learn what may be regarded as socially acceptable behaviour and, in particular, find it difficult to learn responses that are either motivated by fear or reinforced by fear reduction. There is experimental evidence to suggest that psychopaths are correspondingly less able to make connections between past events and the consequentiality of future behaviour.

Long term substance abuse

It should be noted here that the effects of long term substance abuse often bear a close resemblance to severe personality disorder (SPD). Such secondary personality disordered individuals can usually be distinguished from true or primary personality disordered individuals

---

4.   See *Suggestions for Further Reading.*

by the presence of anxiety or guilt in the secondary group. This can normally only be distinguished by highly skilled staff, since the 'psychopathic' individual will demonstrate highly manipulative behaviour, making this distinction hard to make.

The close interrelationship between psychopathy and substance abuse has been acknowledged for some time and issues of co-morbidity are ever present for researchers involved in clinical studies.

A prospective longitudinal study was carried out by Knop *et al* (1993), in which an experimental cohort of 255 children with alcoholic fathers was identified. It followed the children's development until the age of 30. At the conclusion of the study the social functioning of the group with substance dependence and/or anti-social personality disorder was significantly poorer than that of all other diagnostic groups. It may therefore be possible to utilise this type of research to predict those individuals who may be at a higher risk of developing substance abuse disorders and/or anti-social personality disorder later in life. What we do know is that those suffering from it or, perhaps more importantly, making others suffer from it, are extremely difficult to work with and manage (see *Chapter 3*).

Some Further Developments in the Neurosciences

Asperger's syndrome (ASPD) and attention deficit hyperactivity disorder (ADHD).

Asperger's Syndrome

Asperger's syndrome forms part of the broader condition known as Autism Spectrum Disorder (ASPD). It is believed that some 600,000 people in the UK are affected by such disorders. Those suffering from them have impaired capacity to interact with others and problems in 'reading' social situations and responding in an appropriate manner.

Research reported in the *Journal of Neuroscience*[5] indicates that a

---

5.   See the *Independent*, 11 August 2010, p 4.

test has been developed which enables identification of the degree to which sufferers from ASPD have problems in recognising facial expressions as indicators of emotional content. Some confirmation of these findings is also provided in certain work by Professor Stephen Swinderby of the Open University. In a series of laboratory controlled experiments with young sufferers from Asperger's syndrome, he and his colleagues found that their subjects had problems in responding to facial images, but had less difficulty with inanimate objects (Annual Science Lecture entitled 'Imaging the Autistic Brain'—given at Oakham School, Rutland, on 22 February, 2008).

Such findings must be examined with a degree of caution. Professor Paul Matthews of the Centre For Clinical Neurosciences at Imperial College, London[6] considers that 'the findings suggest that sophisticated approaches for the interpretation of brain scans could help to diagnose particular forms of Autistic Spectrum Disorder, although they do not yet offer an approach to confident early diagnosis'.

A further important caveat needs to be entered here. These findings in no way suggest that sufferers from Asperger's syndrome are any more or less likely to be delinquent than non-sufferers. However, rare instances of the connection can occur, as for example, in the case of a York University student who, with an accomplice, was involved in a sophisticated cheating attempt in some examinations. The trial judge told the sufferer that 'I am persuaded that your underlying Asperger's condition has had a marked influence on your poor judgement as to what happened' (as reported in *The Independent*, 1 March, 2008). For studies on the forensic mental health implications of Autism Spectrum Disorder readers may care to consult Deeley *et al* (2006), Murphy (2007) and Tiffin *et al* (2007).

---

6. *Ibid.*

Attention Deficit Hyperactivity Disorder (ADHD)

Research in an allied field, ADHD, has indicated that there may be a genetic basis for such a disorder, thus providing some confirmation for the evidence that the disorder does seem to 'run' in families. As with other forms of disordered or difficult behaviour in children, the parents have all too often been subjected to blame for faulty parenting or, indeed, have blamed themselves. Professor Anita Tharpar, a professor of child and adolescent psychiatry at Cardiff University, and a leader of a relatively recently published study, suggests that 'To manage children with ADHD you need to be a super-parent to handle the difficulties. But that doesn't mean the parenting *caused* the difficulties' (As reported in *The Independent*, 30 September, 2010, p 6, emphasis added).

Neuro-chemistry

The role of neuro-chemistry (as for example in the study of serotonin levels in aggressive behaviour) has developed some prominence. Minzenberg and Siever (in Patrick, 2007) suggest that 'studies [have] consistently demonstrated that aggressive crime and suicidal behaviour were associated with decreased levels of overall activity in the serotonin system' (p 252). Other chemical and hormone systems covered in their review include dopamine, norepinephrine, testosterone, cortisol and thyroid function. The authors stress, however, that research so far into these chemical elements is only at a very early stage.

Neuroanatomy

Raine and Yang (in Patrick, 2007) reviewed some of the important findings in this area through the use of increasingly sophisticated brain imaging analysis (see earlier discussion). They state that

> the key brain areas that have been shown to be abnormal in anti-social individuals include the pre-frontal cortex, temporal cortex, the

amygdala-hippocampal complex, the corpus callosum, and the angular gyrus (p 278).

They also suggest, from a detailed review of the state of research,

that the brain region most likely to be compromised in anti-social, violent populations is the pre-frontal cortex (p 279).

Having made this statement the authors go on to caution against extrapolating too widely at this stage from what are limited exploratory studies.

Family Constellation and Psychopathy

The fathers have eaten sour grapes and the children's teeth are set on edge.

Book of Ezekiel, Chapter 18, verse 2.

Although the main focus in this chapter has been on those physical and organic conditions that may influence the development of serious anti-social (psychopathic) behaviour, I have, from time-to-time, referred to certain psychological 'insults' that may play their part in the complex 'mix' of relevant factors. Before concluding this chapter, I feel it important to refer to one or two long-term studies of delinquent behaviour that add to what has already been said. In an early study, Sheldon and Eleanor Glueck (1962) carried out a large-scale survey of delinquent children in the United States, and Lee Robins (1966) took advantage of the closure of a child guidance clinic to safeguard the clinic's records from incineration. She was able to commence a long-term follow-up of the clinic's patients. It is of interest that she found that children diagnosed with various anxiety type conditions did not go on to become delinquent, but those who were diagnosed as behaviourally disordered did so.

Undoubtedly, one of the most important studies in this field in the UK is that known as 'The Cambridge Study in Delinquent Development' led by Professors Donald West and David Farrington. Farrington (in Patrick, 2007) provides a detailed account of this piece of research which up-dates previous publications. The study covered a 40-year period looking into the histories of children from age eight into adulthood (age 40 plus).

Remarkably, a 93 per cent follow-up rate was achieved. No other study appears to have successfully managed this. West and Farrington (1973, 1976), with their research teams, assessed the influence of family factors under seven categories:

1. Child rearing problems (for example poor supervision, poor discipline, coldness and rejection, low parental involvement with the child);
2. Abuse (physical and sexual) or neglect;
3. Parental conflict and disrupted families;
4. Large family size;
5. Criminal or anti-social parents or siblings;
6. Other characteristics of parents (young age, substance abuse, stress or depression, working mother); and
7. Factors such as low income and poor housing.

Farrington discusses the complex relationship between these different factors and the elements within them that might help to prevent the development of serious anti-social personality in later life. He also stresses the need for the development of effective preventive measures and for research endeavours at an international level. He concludes that such studies should include prospective longitudinal surveys with high risk community samples to investigate the development of psychopathy and the link between psychopathic parents and psychopathic children (p 245).

Concluding Comments

Possible developments in the field are summed up in succinct fashion by Seto and Quinsey in Patrick (2007). They state:

> ... major progress in the near future is likely to be dominated by advances in neuroscience associated with better neuro-imaging technologies, a better understanding of how and where neuro-transmitters work ... the prospects for progress in the treatment of psychopathy are likely similar for the other major conditions such as schizophrenia that are known to be at least partly heritable, to arise during development and to have neurological correlates. Only basic research can provide insight into the aetiology of psychopathy, but such investigations even when successful, require applied and evaluative research to transform the resulting aetiological insights into practical interventions (pp 598-599).

Amen to these views.[7]

Some Further Considerations

The work edited by Patrick mentioned earlier in this chapter provides detailed examination of a number of factors I have alluded to only briefly in the above account. See, for example, in that work Blackburn on social factors, which include tracing the influence of psycho-analytic theory and, more generally, psychodynamic theories, and Harrison Gough's role-taking theory and the capacity to put oneself in the shoes of others showing genuine empathy.

Blackburn concludes his comprehensive survey of the various theoretical stances taken in the last 100 years or so in his statement that:

> 'Despite the claimed contentiousness of the debate over whether psychopathy is a discrete category or the extreme of a continuum, most theories explicitly adopt the latter view' (p 53).

---

7.   See also Cooke et al (2007) and Fowles and Dindo 2007.

One way of demonstrating a possible continuum in terms of progressive seriousness may be seen in *Figure 2* below:

Figure 2: A Progression of Seriousness

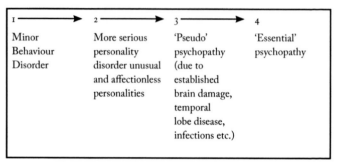

1 →	2 →	3 →	4
Minor Behaviour Disorder	More serious personality disorder unusual and affectionless personalities	'Pseudo' psychopathy (due to established brain damage, temporal lobe disease, infections etc.)	'Essential' psychopathy

Prins, 1980, p.143.

Questions

1. Having read this chapter, what view have you come to in considering psychopathy as an illness?

2. How might advances in the neurosciences impact upon the determination of criminal responsibility (for example, in homicide cases)?

3. Before deciding whether someone's personality is disordered, or severely disordered, what do we really know of what personality is?

Suggestions for Further Reading

The textbook edited by Christopher Patrick is a general source of reference for many of the things discussed in this chapter: see Patrick C. J. (ed.) *Handbook of Psychopathy*. New York: Guilford Press.

Blair *et al*, 2005 for elaboration of dementia and other disorders.

Lyman and Derefinko, 2007 for elaboration of 'dislike' and 'rejection' of psychopaths.

Snowden and Kane, 2003; Tyrer, 1990, Tyrer *et al*, 1990; and Tyrer *et al*, 2003 for further elaboration of the DSMIV and ICD10 tests mentioned under the heading 'What is Personality?'

The *Journal of Forensic Psychiatry and Psychology*, Vol 22(5),October 2011, especially the contribution by Richard C. Howard concerning the role of excitement.

Chapter Three
Aspects of Management

'The history of "psychopathy" begins in the formation of a concept in the minds of philosophers and mad-doctors. Thereafter, the concept becomes linked with a succession of ill-defined terms of art, until one of these is seized upon by legislators and bundled onto the statute-book'.

Walker and McCabe, 1973, p 205.

'Bad laws are the worst form of tyranny'.

Edmund Burke, Speech at Bristol Previous to the Late Election, 1780.

'The notion that convicts are ungovernable is certainly erroneous. There is a mode of managing them with ease to yourself and advantage to them ... manage them with calmness, yet with steadiness'.

John Howard, 1777.

Introduction

In the first two chapters, I made brief reference to some aspects of the management of those labelled as psychopathic. I now consider these in more detail. At the risk of considerable over-simplification, the general history of treatment of the mentally disordered could be summed up by the words *Possession, Containment, Tolerance?*' The question mark after "Tolerance" is deliberate. This is because, despite a considerable degree of progress, there are still serious concerns about the degree of tolerance shown today for the plight of the mentally disordered and the mentally disordered offender in particular.[1] Witness, for example, the obstacles frequently placed in

---

1. The wording is taken from the title of *Chapter 1* in *Signs of Stress: The Social Problems of Psychiatric Illness*, McCulloch and Prins (1978), London: Woburn Press.

the way of those who wish to provide residential facilities (such as hostels) for the last group. Parker summarises some of the historical aspects of the problem.

> 'The practice of confining the insane stretches back over 600 years in England. The type of detained patient has varied, always including those considered to be dangerous. The forms of security have changed little over the period, perimeter security, internal locks and bars and individual restraint by both physical and chemical means have been in continuous use to a greater or lesser degree in various guises up to the present day'.
>
> Parker, 1985:15.[2]

In *Figure 3* I have provided a summary of the general methods for dealing with the mentally disordered through the courts, criminal justice and penal systems. Such provisions would include services for those deemed to be suffering from 'psychopathic' disorder; though, as mentioned earlier in this book the label no longer features in current mental health legislation. A study of history also teaches us that to be both 'mad' and 'bad' places those so designated at the bottom end of the social priority pecking order; these are the 'people that nobody owns' (see Prins, 1993 for further discussion). There is another important consequence of this attitude, namely that those who work with such 'ownerless' individuals may themselves come to feel alienated and contaminated and, as such, may be exposed to prejudicial attitudes (fanned by the less responsible media) as are their patients/clients. This is particularly likely to be the case with those offenders showing psychopathic characteristics.

From as early as the 18th century some provision existed for those who were considered both mad *and dangerous*. However, it was not until the 19th century that special measures were introduced

---

2.   See also *Suggestions for Further Reading* at the end of this chapter.

Figure 3: Outline disposal of mentally disordered offenders through the criminal justice, forensic mental health and penal systems.

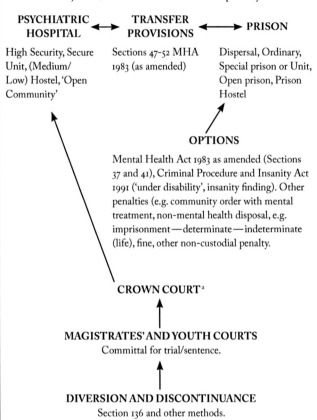

PSYCHIATRIC HOSPITAL ←→ **TRANSFER PROVISIONS** ←→ **PRISON**

High Security, Secure Unit, (Medium/ Low) Hostel, 'Open Community'	Sections 47-52 MHA 1983 (as amended)	Dispersal, Ordinary, Special prison or Unit, Open prison, Prison Hostel

OPTIONS

Mental Health Act 1983 as amended (Sections 37 and 41), Criminal Procedure and Insanity Act 1991 ('under disability', insanity finding). Other penalties (e.g. community order with mental treatment, non-mental health disposal, e.g. imprisonment—determinate—indeterminate (life), fine, other non-custodial penalty.

CROWN COURT[a]

MAGISTRATES' AND YOUTH COURTS
Committal for trial/sentence.

DIVERSION AND DISCONTINUANCE
Section 136 and other methods.

Notes

a   The powers available to the Crown Court are also exercisable on appeal by the Court of Appeal.

b   Magistrates may also commit to the Crown Court with a view to a hospital order being made *with restrictions*.

c   This figure and some of the following material are taken from Prins, 2010 and it is reproduced here by kind permission of the publishers.

d   See *Chapter 4* for further elaboration of the statutory position.

for the *public* as well as for the private care and treatment of mentally disordered individuals; and doubtless these would have included a proportion of those who, today, would be designated as psychopathic.[3]

Some would have found their way into the prisons, as John Howard discovered during his classic investigation into *The State of the Prisons* (1777). Others, no doubt, would have found their way into such institutions as the houses of correction or bridewells, or would have even suffered public execution or transportation.

The early 20th century witnessed a trend to introduce legislation designed to make available provision for those who not only showed criminal behaviour, but also exhibited varying degrees of what was then described as 'idiocy' or 'mental deficiency'. The Mental Deficiency Act of 1913 permitted courts to deal more effectively with such offenders by enabling them to be taken out of the penal system and placed in hospital care. Such provision which, at the time, may have seemed humane, often led to unfortunate consequences. For example, it stressed the notion of moral degeneracy (derived, no doubt, from the influence of the eugenics movement); for example, it linked female promiscuity with mental deficiency. This led to a number of women who had given birth to illegitimate children being labelled as 'moral defectives' or 'moral imbeciles'[4] and

---

3.   For example, in the 18th century the mentally disordered could be found in the following types of accommodation and their treatment at this time was frequently based largely upon superstition, moral condemnation, ignorance and apathy. There were patients confined:

   1.   Under the Poor Law.
   2.   Under the criminal law.
   3.   Under various Vagrancy Acts perhaps the best-known of which is that of 1824.
   4.   In private madhouses.
   5.   As Bethlem (Bedlam) patients.
   6.   As 'single lunatics', i.e. in private houses, often under the most appalling conditions.

   See also *Suggestions for Further Reading* at the end of this chapter.

4.   In addition to such terms, the law introduced 'idiocy' and

made them liable perhaps to life-long detention in secure hospitals.[5]

Later Legislation

The Mental Health Act 1959

The 1959 Act developed from the Report of the *Royal Commission on Mental Illness and Mental Deficiency* (1957). This report had recommended three groups of patients:

- the higher-grade feeble-minded and moral defectives and other 'psychopathic' patients. They suggested that these should be classified as a main group of mentally disordered patients;
- the mentally ill; and
- the severely subnormal.

In respect of the psychopathic group, these were to be distinguished from the severely subnormal by virtue of their showing abnormally aggressive or inadequate social behaviour. The commission recommended the use of the words 'psychopathic patients' and 'psychopathic personality'.

When the Act became law in 1959, four groupings were identified, i.e. concerning those affected by:

- mental illness (not further defined);
- mental subnormality;
- severe mental subnormality; and
- psychopathy.

'feeble-mindedness'. It was not until the late-1950s that these terms were to disappear from statute.

5.   History reveals that there had been a longstanding attempt to distinguish between 'madmen' and 'natural fools' (fatuoram naturaliam). Idiocy seems to have been recognised as a permanent condition and madness as a temporary state (see Walker, 1968; and Walker and McCabe, 1973).

The 1959 Act was considered to be ground-breaking at the time. It swept away the complex legal provisions of the Lunacy Act 1890,[6] the Mental Deficiency Acts of 1913 and 1927 and the Mental Treatment Act 1930. The emphasis was to be on informal, that is non-compulsory, hospital admission. Safeguards were introduced in respect of patients requiring the latter and the introduction of further safeguards in the guise of the Mental Health Review Tribunal (MHRT) to see that patients (including offender-patients) were appropriately detained.

In addition, the 1959 Act made provision for the courts to make, in appropriate cases, hospital orders and to add an order for restricting the discharge of offender-patients thought to be dangerous (sections 60/65).

Under the 1959 Act, the Mental Health Review Tribunal could only *recommend* discharge of restricted patients to the Home Secretary. This was to change under the provisions of the 1983 Act (see below). The 1959 Act defined psychopathy as a 'persistent disorder of disability of [the] mind (whether or not including subnormality of intelligence) and [that] requires or is susceptible to treatment'. This formulation was to engender much concern as to what constituted treatment and about the implied links between mental subnormality and criminality (see further below).

There had been a considerable degree of dissatisfaction with various aspects of the 1959 Act. A major concern had been the notion of 'treatability', *particularly in respect of those designated as psychopathic*. There had also been concern about the more general treatment of detained patients.

---

6. Some idea of the complex and cumbersome nature of the Lunacy Act 1890 may be gained from the table at *Appendix 2* attached to the *Report of the Royal Commission on Mental Illness and Mental Deficiency* (1957). It measures two feet six inches across by 15 inches down and it also has 17 columns across and nine down!

Mental Health Act 1983

A number of measures were introduced in order to deal with these matters. MHRTs were given the power to *order* the discharge of restricted offender-patients provided certain strict criteria were satisfied, particularly those pertaining to the risk of further dangerous offending. Panels hearing such appeals were to be chaired by either a senior barrister or a Crown Court judge.

The 1983 Act introduced a treatability test. For detention (or renewal) of the section, the authorised doctor under the Act had to 'verify that medical treatment was likely to alleviate or prevent a deterioration in the patient's condition. This would be hard to do if the patient was resolutely not co-operating ... treatment might be available and appropriate but unlikely to make any difference if the patient refused to co-operate' (Fennell, 2007, p 67). 'The 2007 Act [see below] only requires that treatment be available, regardless of whether the patient accepts' (p 67).

An important innovation under the 1983 Act had been provision for a Mental Health Act Commission to deal with complaints from detained patients. It also provided for a Code of Practice—to be revised and up-dated at regular intervals.

Mental Health Act 2007

Over the years, interpretations of certain sections of the 1983 Act led to their determination by various judicial bodies, such as the European Court of Human Rights (ECHR) the Court of Appeal and, subsequently, through the Human Rights Act 1998.

Concern had also developed because of the offending activities of a small number of patients and offender-patients, and a conclusion on the part of one central government minister, that community care had failed. Much of this concern was fuelled by the less responsible media; two examples being the entry of a patient—Ben Silcock—into the lions' enclosure at the London Zoo and Michael Fagin's intrusion into the Queen's bedroom at Buckingham Palace. Perhaps even more important was the wider development of a 'moral panic' (Cohen, 2007) thrown up by the commission of a small number of homicides by those having had past and/or current contact with the mental health and allied services, one of the most notable being the activities of Michael Stone (whose case is discussed later in this chapter).

In the light of some of these and other events, the then Secretary of State for Health ordered, in somewhat peremptory fashion, a 'root and branch' review of the 1983 Act. The remit, when announced, was both highly proscriptive and prescriptive.

Against this somewhat limiting background, the Review Committee, under the skilled chairmanship of Professor Genevra Richardson, produced a most thoughtful report (1999). It stressed the need for any future Act to include 'balancing' principles between individual rights and public safety. The committee's report appears to have been somewhat brusquely ignored by government, who went on to produce, in speedy fashion, Green and White Papers. Professor Jill Peay, who had been a member of the committee, rightly described the government's response as a 'squandered opportunity' (Peay, 2000). At a later stage the government produced its famous (or infamous, depending upon your ethical viewpoint) policy paper on the politically generated diagnosis of dangerous and severe personality disorder (DSPD) (see later).

Over the last two or three decades there appears to have been an increasing degree of illiberality towards mental health patients in general and offender-patients in particular (see Grounds, 2001 for elaboration of this important aspect). These views were quite evident in the formulation of two abortive Mental Health Bills, which received a considerable mauling during the parliamentary process. This suggests an analogy akin to that ascribed to marriage — 'legislate in haste, repent at leisure'.

The 2007 Act received the Royal Assent in July of that year. Some of the most relevant provisions for our purposes can be summarised as follows:

- The former classification and definitions of mental disorder were replaced by an all-embracing definition—thus mental disorder now means 'any disorder or disability of mind'.

- At last, the term 'psychopathy' disappears; in addition, the contentious treatability clauses which appeared in different guises in the 1959 and 1983 Mental Health Acts are replaced by 'appropriate medical treatment' (being available).

- There is a new definition of 'medical treatment'. This now consists of 'psychological intervention and specialist mental health habilitation, rehabilitation and care, the purpose of which is to alleviate, or prevent worsening of the disorder, or one or more of its symptoms or manifestations'. It is interesting to note that the word 'alleviation', which was in the 1983 Act, is retained. In a recent contribution, Phull and Bartlett (2012) make a number of criticisms concerning the lack of further detail about the use of the term 'appropriate treatment' in the 2007 Act. They quote at some length three cases that provide evidence for their own conclusions that a fuller definition and explanation of that term is needed. They suggest that any future cases referred for review by the 'Upper Tribunal' and/or the High Court may indicate that the term may require legislative amendment and elucidation.

- Various sections of the 2007 Act permit a broadening of the range of professionals who can now exercise powers under it. For example, the designation 'approved social worker' (ASW) is replaced by 'approved mental health professional' (AMHP). This

enables a wide range of professionals to perform former ASW functions. For example, nurses, occupational
therapists and chartered psychologists.

- One of the most controversial provisions of the Act
  is the power to make community treatment orders.
  These permit patients, already detained under the Act,
  to be discharged subject to specific conditions, and
  made liable to be recalled to hospital if these have been
  infringed. These new powers can be seen as a 'beefing
  up' of the provisions (now abandoned) for supervised
  discharge orders (after-care under supervision) under
  the Mental Health (Patients in the Community) Act
  1995. Appeals against community treatment orders are
  dealt with by the MHTs.

- The Act makes certain changes in organization and
  nomenclature to the MHT system. The pre-existing
  multiple tribunals for England are replaced by one tribunal under the direction of a president (Wales already
  had a presidential arrangement). Hitherto known
  as presidents of individual tribunals, they are now
  known as chairmen. Tribunals now come under the
  jurisdiction of the Ministry of Justice; previously they
  had been under the jurisdiction of the Department of
  Health.[7]

- The longstanding practice of allowing restriction
  orders to be made with a limit of time, is replaced by
  indefinite orders. This change acknowledges that the

---

7.   Although they will continue to be known by most people as MHRTs the
     nomenclature has become more complicated. As Mental Health Tribunals
     (MHTs) they now form part of the First Tier Tribunals as an element of
     the Health and Social Care 'Chamber' (see Gledhill, 2009, for details).

assessment of risk should not be impeded by a finite
period of detention.

• Schedule 6 of the 2007 Act allows victims of certain
  offences of violence, or of a sexual nature, the same
  rights as those exercisable under the Domestic Violence, Crime and Victims Act 2004. This provision
  enables representations to be made by victims or their
  representatives relating to the proposed discharge of
  unrestricted offender-patients.[8]

Close Encounters of an Uncomfortable Kind

'Listen to me, but do listen, and let that be the comfort you offer me.
Bear with me while I have my say'.

Book of Job, 21, 2-3, *New English Bible*.

From what I have written so far, I hope it has become obvious that
those labelled as 'psychopathic' present considerable psycho-so-
cio-legal problems and that their day-to-day management causes
the professionals involved both 'headache' and 'heartache'. Certain
aspects of mental health and criminal justice professionals' engage-
ment in these 'encounters' have already been touched upon; and
my intention in what follows is merely to highlight some of them
further.

The late Dr Peter Scott addressed some of these issues over 30
years ago in a thought-provoking but under-referred-to-paper entitled 'Has Psychiatry Failed in the Treatment of Offenders?' (1975).
Scott suggested that we most frequently fail those who need us most.
Such individuals often fall into two (perhaps overlapping) categories: the 'dangerous offender'; and the 'unrewarding', 'degenerate'
and 'not nice' offender.

---

8. For further elaboration of this short account, see Fennell (2007).

Of such 'embarrassing' patients, Scott (1975:8) maintained that he/she is the patient who is

> ... essentially the one who does not pay for treatment, the coin in which the patient pays being (i) dependence — i.e. being manifestly unable to care for themselves, and thus appealing to the maternal part of our nature; (ii) getting better (responding to our 'life-giving' measures); (iii) in either of these processes, showing gratitude, if possible cheerfully.

In other words, those patients/clients/offenders that Scott had in mind are the ones who reject our 'best efforts'; they are manipulative, and delight in giving us a pretext for rejecting them so that they can continue on their 'unloved' and 'unloving' way. In Scott's terms, 'the "not nice" patients' are the ones who

> habitually appear to be well able to look after themselves but don't, and [as stated above] reject attempts to help them, break institutional rules, get drunk, upset other patients, or even quietly go to the devil in their own way quite heedless of nurse and doctor.

Scott went on to suggest other factors which are relevant to any consideration of the management of *so-called* psychopaths. I emphasise the word 'so-called' because Scott did not feel there was much merit in distinguishing psychopaths from hardened chronic (recidivist) criminals — albeit a minority view (Scott 1960). In support of this, he advocated that such individuals would be best dealt with in specialist units within the prison system. He also stated (1975:9) that:

> 'There is a natural philanthropic tendency to extend help to the defenceless — probably an extension of parental caring ... if this fails so that embarrassing people or patients are seen to accumulate, then anxiety is aroused and some form of institution is set up to absorb the problem ... Not all embarrassing patients like being

tidied up and these tend to be compulsorily detained ... Within
the detaining institution two opposing aims begin to appear—the
therapeutic endeavour to cure and liberate on the one hand, and
the controlling custodial function on the other'.

He also considered that although these functions should be com-
plimentary 'there is a tendency for them to polarise and ultimately,
to split, like a dividing cell, into two separate institutions' (Scott
1975:10). However, he also made the point that

neither of the two new institutions can quite eliminate the tendency
from which it fled, so that the therapeutic institution now begins
to miss the custodial function and tries hard to send some of its
patients back to custody, and the custodial institution is unable to
tolerate being unkind to people all the time and begins to set up a
new nucleus of therapy.

His perceptive 'management' observations have in some respects
been taken on board by those involved in implementing the institutional care programme for DSPD individuals (see later). These are
the unlikeable clients/patients/offenders and sometimes this dislike
will operate at an unconscious level. Three, admittedly somewhat
'dated', quotations of the views of psychiatrists are useful in illustrat-
ing this problem; their words are also applicable to all professionals
working in the field of criminal justice and forensic mental health.
For example, Maier (1990, p 776) suggested:

'Could it be after all these Freudian years, that psychiatrists have
denied the hatred they feel for psychopaths and criminals, and thus
have been unable to treat psychopaths adequately because their
conceptual bases for treatment have been distorted by unconscious,
denied feelings from the start?'

A somewhat similar view had been proffered earlier by

Treves-Brown (1977:63), who stated that:

> 'As long as a doctor believes that psychopaths are mostly "bad", his
> successful treatment rate will be dismal. Since it takes two to form
> a relationship, an outside observer could be forgiven for suspecting
> that a doctor who describes a patient as unable to form a relation-
> ship, is simply trying to justify his own hostility to his patient'.

Winnicott (1949:71) — a doyen of child psychiatry, writing over
half a century ago about the 'anti-social' tendency — gave further
support for such views as follows:

> 'However much he loves his ... [hard to like] ... patients he cannot
> help hating them and fearing them, and the better he knows this
> the less will hate and fear be the motives determining what he does
> for his patients.

Interestingly, at about the same time as Winnicott was writing, another psychoanalytically orientated psychiatrist — Melitta
Schmideberg — was describing (somewhat provocatively) the extent
to which applied psychoanalysis could also be combined with providing practical help to serious offenders.

This view did not endear her to many of her professional
colleagues (see Schmideberg, 1949). The volume in which her contribution appears offers an excellent review of what psychoanalytic
principles might offer to the understanding of delinquent behaviour
in the late-1940s and early-1950s.

These statements indicate that the mechanism of 'denial' is not
merely the prerogative of patients and offenders.

Despite the unattractiveness of psychopathic patients and the
sometimes unconscious rejecting reactions of therapists, a number of forensic mental health and criminal justice professionals
have expressed a degree of optimism about treatment. Some years
ago Tennent *et al* (1993) sought the opinions of psychiatrists,

psychologists and probation officers about treatability. Admittedly, the survey was small, as was the response rate. However, there was reasonable evidence to suggest that although there were few clear-cut views as to the best treatment modalities, there *were* also clear indications as to those felt to be helpful. For example, there were higher expectations of treatment efficacy with symptoms such as 'chronically anti-social', 'abnormally aggressive' and 'lacking control impulses' and much lower expectations for symptoms such as 'inability to experience guilt', 'lack of remorse or shame' and 'pathological egocentricity'.

Support for the findings of this modest survey can be found in a much more extensive one by Cope (1993) on behalf of the Forensic Section of the Royal College of Psychiatrists. Cope surveyed all forensic psychiatrists working in secure hospitals, units and similar settings in England and Wales. The majority of her respondents (response rate 91%) were in favour of offering treatment to severely personality disordered (psychopathic) patients. Some confirmation of this optimism derives from another source.

In an attempt to ascertain the motivations of consultant forensic psychiatrists for working in forensic psychiatric settings, the present author discovered that one of the attractions of the work was the challenge presented by 'psychopaths' (Prins, 1998). Another fact that emerged from this survey was the need for forensic psychiatrists to work with and encourage their colleagues in general psychiatry to deal with such patients—a point emphasised cogently by Gunn (1999). He suggests that 'someone has to deal' with such individuals and psychiatry should play its full part.[9]

Some statements by a number of the present author's respondents were illuminating. One of them enjoyed the challenge presented by the severity and complexity of the cases which produced 'a kind of appalled fascination'. Another attraction was the chance to work with a wide range of agencies and disciplines and to pursue a more

---

9. See also the *Suggestions for Further Reading* at the end of this chapter.

eclectic approach to patient care. Stimulation was another important factor, One respondent stated

> 'I could not envisage 20 years of listening to the neurotic and wor-
> ried well ... after forensic psychiatry, other specialities [within the
> field] seemed very tame and had much less variety and challenge'.

Whatever form of professional training is eventually formulated
in order to deal more effectively with psychopathically disordered
individuals, understanding and management will only be successful through the adoption of the need for a truly multi-disciplinary
approach (as implied in the 'imaginary' gathering described towards
the end of *Chapter 1* of this book).

Such an approach would not only serve to take the broadest possible view of the topic but, at a narrower clinical level, should help
to obviate potential missed diagnoses (for example, the importance
of organic factors such as brain damage). Scott (1960, p 1645) had
some interesting observations to make on this matter. He stated that:

> 'This may be the point at which to acknowledge that, with psy-
> chopaths, highly refined psychotherapeutic procedures applied by
> medical men, are often no more successful, sometimes less success-
> ful, than the simpler and less esoteric approaches of certain social
> workers, probation officers [and others] ... some workers intuitively
> obtain good results with certain psychopaths; it should be possible
> to find out how they do it ... (See also Schmideberg, 1949).

Sadly, no definitive research information is available to answer
Scott's question about treatment success. However, what we do
know is that severely dangerous and deviant behaviour requires
calm and well-informed confrontation. In the words of the late
George Lyward—a highly gifted worker with severely personality
disordered older adolescents—'Patience is love that can wait' (see
Burn, 1956 for elaboration).

Coupled with this is the need to tolerate, without loss of temper, the hate, hostility, manipulation and 'splitting' shown by such individuals, together with an ability not to take such personal affronts as attacks. The psychiatrist and psychotherapist Penelope Campling (1996) has provided an excellent account of the management of such behaviours within a therapeutic community unit.[10]

It is also essential for professionals to have more than an 'intellectual' understanding of what the patient has done. Sometimes, this can be 'stomach-churning' and offers many opportunities for denial on the part of the professional. Such understanding also requires a degree of what has been described in another context as 'intestinal fortitude', an expression used by Michael Davies, Leader of the BBC Symphony Orchestra, in relation to the playing of certain problematical orchestral works (BBC broadcast, 10 July 1999).

It is worth re-emphasising the importance of the phenomenon of denial which is not the sole prerogative of clients/patients/offenders. For, as Pericles says in Shakespeare's play of that name,

'Few love to hear the sins they love to act' (Act I, Scene 1).

For example, in some instances a mental health or criminal justice professional may ignore an individual's underlying past vulnerability because their current behaviour horrifies them due to its very malignancy.

In *Chapter 1,* I made brief reference to the role of applied psychoanalytic techniques in the understanding of serious (particularly violent) offending. I can recall how evident this was in my training as a probation officer in the early-1950s. Many of the lecturing inputs from psychiatrists were from those with a psychoanalytic bias. In addition, some of the inputs from our tutors were based upon many of the same principles, much of which stemmed from the influence of American social work teachers who had been schooled

---

10. See also Suggestions for Further Reading at the end of this chapter.

in the practice of child guidance which had similar origins. Many of these influences seemed to fade in subsequent years and be overtaken by behaviourist principles and practice.

There has been a 'swing' back again to the espousal of applied psychoanalytic principles and practice, and particularly those stemming from classical Freudian and post-Freudian approaches. These are well illustrated in a compilation of contributions edited by Gordon and Kirtchuk. The book's title *Psychic Assaults and Frightened Clinicians* (2008) gives the 'flavour' of what they are trying to convey. Readers should note here that the insights adumbrated in the book are psychoanalytic *derivatives*; the editors and their various authors are not suggesting that the formal practice of classical psychoanalytic techniques are applicable, merely that the insights *derived* from its practice may be helpful in understanding the traumatic origins of seriously deviant behaviour (particularly offences of a seriously sexual and violent nature).

In their editorial introduction to the book the authors stress the importance of a number of psychoanalytic concepts and, in particular, that of *countertransference*—as follows:

> The unconscious effect of the worker's feelings, thoughts and behaviours of the patient's symptoms, actions, history, communications and impacts.

The title of the book includes the words 'psychic assaults' to convey the often shocking collision which underlies a simple meeting between two people, a patient and a staff member (p 3).

They indicate the need to take on board insights suggested above—as follows:

> 'In clinical work with forensic patients who are themselves out of touch with what has happened in their lives (both to themselves and to others) the worker's awareness of his or her feelings is often

the main vehicle for understanding the patient's emotional states, psychopathology and offending behaviours' (p3).

It should be noted that over the last three decades or so there has been what might perhaps be described as a 'rebirth' of interest and practice in using these derivatives.

There are now courses in forensic mental health psychotherapy, which utilise such concepts; and the early-1990s saw the inauguration of the International Association for Forensic Psychotherapy. This body has brought together many of the leading practitioners in the field. I emphasise that the applied psychoanalytic approach fostered by the association in no way supplants a more behavioural approach, such as cognitive behavioural therapy (CBT) and its derivatives.

A further concept allied to counter-transference is that of 'projective identification' (originated in the work of Melanie Klein). It is described by Ayegbusi and Tuck (in Gordon and Kirtchuk (2008) (see also Gordon, *et al* 2008)) as 'a very primitive method—often the only possible one—of expressing unmanageable feelings by locating them in others rather than in oneself' (p 16).[11] The more troublesome and anxiety-making the relationship, the more the need not to go it alone. This is not an area of work that should be characterised by 'prima donna' activities by professionals of either sex, for there are dangerous workers as well as dangerous clients/patients/offenders.

In my view, there are three qualities that are of paramount importance in dealing with severely personality (psychopathically) disordered individuals. These are:

- *Consistence* The capacity to take a firm line in dealing with deflecting activities by the offender;

---

11. See also *Suggestions for Further Reading* at the end of this chapter.

- *Persistence* Expending efforts over very considerable periods of time, perhaps even years—a view that is supported by the belief in the occurrence of cortical maturation and the longer term benefits of team therapy in institutions such as those at Grendon Prison described by Taylor (2000) and Coughlin (2003). Put in more vernacular terms, the capacity to 'hang in there'; and finally,

- *Insistence* The capacity to give clear indications that requirements of supervision are to be met in spite of resistance on the part of the offender. Such insistence must take priority when expectations of what supervision requires of the offender are initially set out in the professional/client relationship.[12]

An Australian Illustration

The problems of trying to *legislate* for persons suffering from severe personality (psychopathic) disorder which may, from time to time, make them a danger to themselves and to others, are exemplified in the extraordinary Australian case of Gary David as told by Deirdre Greig in her disturbing book, *Neither Bad nor Mad* (2002). Her account demonstrates the inability of both the criminal justice and forensic mental healthcare systems to deal with such individuals, and his story may be told here briefly.

Vignette

Gary was born in November 1954 and had a disturbed family history. He died of severe complications arising from grievous self-inflicted injuries in June 1992. Gary's severe personality disorder gave rise to many years of dramatic and highly persistent disruptive and

---

12. See also *Suggestions for Further Reading* at the end of this chapter.

manipulative behaviours. These included serious and highly bizarre episodes of both self-harm and harm to others.

The inability of both systems to deal with Gary effectively led to numerous political manoeuvres to affect his indeterminate detention on the basis of his 'dangerousness'. This included the passing of a single piece of legislation to deal solely with his case.

Over the years, numerous psychiatric professionals who had dealings with him could not agree on the nature and extent of his mental disorder or, in fact, whether or not he was mentally disordered at all.

Limitations of space preclude a detailed discussion of the sad saga of the various commissions of inquiry, court hearings and appeals that dealt with Gary's case, but what they do confirm is the highly complex nature of the fluctuating relationships between health care and penal institutions as described by Scott earlier in this chapter.

One of the more important (but unsurprising) findings in Greig's account (2002, p 151) is suggested by one of her sources of information:

One lesson to be learned from legal history is that hard cases make bad law and that there is a risk that a hasty and ill-conceived response to one particular case … can seriously disturb a larger and well thought out structure.

English central government is much concerned about 'Managing Dangerous People with Severe Personality Disorder' and has sponsored various possibilities, the most disquieting being the *apparent* possibility of detaining someone on the basis of what it is felt *they might do*. Another serious weakness includes the somewhat naïve expectations on the part of politicians that criminal justice and forensic mental health professionals have foolproof skills in predicting future behaviour and its risks. At present, we are trying to treat/manage a very problematic group of people with serious gaps in our knowledge base, coupled with a significant lack of capacity for self-examination when trying to engage with such people. As stated earlier, confronting one's own 'demons' is crucial in this respect. Psychopathic disorder is not going to go away whatever we call the condition in the future; and it has been rightly described as the 'Achilles Heel' of criminal justice and psychiatry.

The Michael Stone Case and DSPD

I have already made brief reference to the case of Michael Stone. I now consider his case in slightly more detail because it can be seen as an important 'generating' factor in the move to introduce the concept of dangerous and severe personality disorder and the provisions developed for its management. The details of what follows are paraphrased mainly from the Court of Appeal's judgement of January 21st 2005 ((2005) EWCA Crim 105, No 200300595/B3).

> On July 9th, 1996, Dr Lin Russell, together with her six-year-old daughter Megan and her older sister Josie, attended a local swimming gala and then began to walk home with the family dog. At about 4.15 pm they were attacked by a man getting out of a car, seemingly intent on robbery (Dr Russell had neither purse nor handbag with her). He took them into a thicket, tied them up with torn towels and shoe laces, blindfolded them, and savagely beat the head of each of them with a hammer, smashing their skulls to a 'greater or lesser degree'.

> Dr Russell and Megan both died. Josie, though very grievously injured, happily survived. The dog was killed. There was no further reference to the killing of the dog. One can only speculate about the motive. Perhaps the dog went to the rescue of the victims, perhaps it was killed before it could run loose and contribute to an alarm

being raised; perhaps there was some deeper psychopathological motive. We just do not know.

In July 1997 (a year after the murders), Michael Stone was arrested and charged with the killings. He went on trial at Maidstone Crown Court in October, 1998, charged with two counts of murder and one of attempted murder. He was convicted on all counts and sentenced to life imprisonment. Stone lodged an immediate appeal and, in February 2001, the Court of Appeal overturned the convictions and ordered a retrial. This took place at Nottingham Crown Court in Autumn 2001. He was convicted afresh and returned to prison to serve his life sentence.

In April 2003, Stone's legal advisers lodged a further appeal, but it was dismissed by the Court of Appeal in January 2005, and leave to appeal to the House of Lords (on the grounds of points of law of general public importance) was refused. Stone's case is of interest, not just for the reasons already stated, but because of the number of trials that took place (For detailed discussion of the subsequent belated homicide inquiry see Prins, 2007, and Francis, 2007).

What Followed

Largely as a result of the Stone case, and some of the other cases referred to earlier in this chapter, four units were established to deal with those adjudged to be suffering (and making others suffer) from DSPD. The uncertainties as to which services seemed best placed to deal with such offenders are reflected perhaps in the decision to split the four units equally between penal and forensic mental health care. Put somewhat crudely, the criteria for inclusion in the DSPD programme were:

(a)   The individual should have a severe personality disorder; and

(b) be deemed to be more likely than not to behave in a manner that would cause serious psychological or physical harm from which the victim would find it difficult or impossible to recover; and

(c) the risk of re-offending should be linked to the personality disorder (see also Barrett *et al*, 2009).

Two of the units are currently prison based (HMP Whitemoor and HMP Frankland) and two are at high security hospitals (Broadmoor and Rampton). A unit for the small number of women DSPD offenders has also been opened at HMP Low Newton.

In addition, a number of medium secure units have developed facilities for personality disordered offenders.

The success or otherwise of these highly specialised facilities has been the subject of much professional debate. Overall, it appears that the consensus as to their cost-effectiveness has been somewhat critical.

Burns *et al* reviewed the various forms of treatment available within the four centres. They concluded that

'A rigorous rationalisation of the treatments is needed to permit a robust evaluation of their effectiveness. Further research is needed to determine whether reductions in risk reflect re-offending rates' (2011, p. 411).

Tyrer *et al* reviewed progress over a ten-year period (following the inception of the programme) and concluded that 'although much has been gained from the experiment — particularly in developing services for those with personality disorder in general — it has been less effective in managing those whom it was primarily targeting and may not have been cost effective' (2010, p 95).

A study by Trebilcock and Weaver (2012) revealed that some MHRT members were sceptical about the ability of DSPD patients to change, and criticised the DSPD programme on the basis that it was 'expensive, politically-motivated and delivering non-evidence based treatments with a low probability of positive outcomes' (p 250). And a further study by the same authors (2012) found that 'a proportion of patients were [being] preventively detained within the DSPD Hospital Units' (p 237). The authors suggest that the DSPD programme be renamed The Personality Disorder Pathway 'in order to develop the capacity to manage more high risk offenders with personality disorder within criminal justice settings' (p 238).[13]

Concluding Comments

I have emphasised in this chapter that the group of people I identify as 'psychopathic' arouse strong emotions in those who are charged with managing them. Discussion about these troubled and troubling individuals often tends to generate more 'heat' than 'light'; I trust that the somewhat brief observations in this chapter will aid more considered discussion. The degree of success (or otherwise) of the four pilot DSPD centres (listed above) will be followed with much interest.

Bowers *et al* (2005) have begun to identify some of the difficulties facing staff and an encouraging sign of the move to more 'joined up working' may be found in a paper by Sizmur and Noutch (2005).[14]

---

13. See also *Suggestions for Further Reading* at the end of this chapter.

14. One of the problems in dealing with high risk offenders, especially those suffering from psychopathic disorder, has been co-operation and collaboration between the various agencies involved. Some years ago, Multi-agency Public Protection Arrangements (MAPPAs) were introduced. These were not functioning as well as had been expected. To deal with this deficiency, revised arrangements were introduced requiring police, probation and prison services to co-operate on a more formal level, through the Criminal Justice and Courts Services Act 2000. For a useful contribution see Henson and Riordan (2012). The Criminal Justice Act 2003 includes an indeterminate sentence for public protection (ISPP) for persons over the age of 18 convicted of a serious offence who pose a significant risk to the public (see Greenall, 2009; Sheldon and Krishnan, 2009; and note that this is under review). All references to probation work is to that under the auspices of the National Probation Service (NPS): see the *Glossary*. There are controversial plans to privatise aspects of probation provision. These

In my opinion, Professor Gunn (1999, pp 75-76) has provided what is a useful and critical summary of the work which still needs to be done.

'In England and Wales we have an uphill struggle on our hands. We need to persuade our Home Office [now Ministry of Justice] not to drop its interest [and I would add to this the Department of Health] and particularly [the] resource allocation for a needy, hitherto neglected group of patients, but at the same time to back away from new types of ... preventive detention laws and focus instead on the well-tried arrangements we already have. It is true that our prisons can do with more psychiatric resources, we have secure hospitals that also need more resources ... we certainly do not need new and restrictive laws. The United Kingdom has many laws which can be used imaginatively if we have sufficient and appropriate staffs. Politicians, many of whom are lawyers, rush to legislate; we need to provide them with resources'.

---

plans are a continuation of current activities to minimise the role of probation staff. This is having a serious impact on morale within the service.

Questions

1. In the light of the content of this chapter, which management regime (prison or hospital) would seem to you to be the most appropriate for someone suffering from the various conditions described?

2. What are the pros and cons of managing people with mental health problems in the community?

3. Given that the assessment of risk is a mix of fact (the existence of circumstances giving rise to concern) and opinion (that of trained professionals: medical and judicial) balanced by the rights of individuals, what level of risk should the public be expected to tolerate?

4. How far have we come from the days of Bedlam and before?

Suggestions for Further Reading

Further details in the *Select Bibliography.*

Adshead, G. and Jacob, C (eds) (2009), *Personality Disorder: The Definitive Reader.* (A useful compilation of published papers).

Department of Health and Ministry of Justice (2010), *Procedure For the Transfer of Prisoners to and from Hospitals Under Sections 47 and 48 of the Mental Health Act, 1983.*

Shaw, J, Minoudis, P, Hamilton, V. A., and Craissati, J. (2012) 'An Investigation into Competency for Working With Personality Disorder in the Probation Service', *Probation Journal: The Journal of Community and Criminal Justice,* 59: 39-48.

Also the August issue (23, No 4) of *The Journal of Forensic Psychiatry and Psychology* contains several papers germane to this chapter.

For those readers wishing to explore the history of incarcerating the insane further, a useful starting point would be the well documented and readable account by the historian Catharine Arnold — *Bedlam: London and Its Mad* (2008).

For studies of work specifically with DSPD patients from the psychiatrists' point of view, see Haddock *et al* (2001), Duggan (2007) and Langton (2007), and from a forensic nursing perspective see Bowers (2002).

For a recent short but cogent account of the various issues involved in determining the future see Taylor (2012).

For an early detailed account of the problem of women giving birth to illegitimate children and use of the term 'moral imbecility', see the

Report of the Royal Commission on the Care and Control of the Feeble Minded (Radnor Commission 1908); and also Lindsay *et al*, 2011.

For a small-scale study of the problems involved in providing services for a 'cluster' of personality disordered patients see Lee *et al* (2008).

For a complementary contribution concerning the use of reflection with forensic mental health patients, see Ferrito *et al*, 2012.

For modern research-based exposition of the potential value of psychosocial therapy for severe personality disorders, see Chiesa and Fonagy (2003).

For useful short accounts of the day-to-day problems involved in the management of DSPD offenders see, for example Sheldon and Tennent (2011) and Sheldon and Krishman (2009), and, more generally, Wilmot and Gordon (eds.) (2011).

Chapter Four
Services and Procedures — Further Considered

In *Chapter 3, Figure 3* sets out the 'bare bones' of the provisions for mentally disordered offenders (which would include the psychopathic). For the benefit of those readers who are unfamiliar with what is a somewhat a complicated system of disposals, I have endeavoured to put some 'flesh' on bones in this chapter. Readers may wish to ignore the anatomical analogy!

Hospital Disposals

Hospital orders
A hospital order lasts initially for six months, is renewable for a further six months and is then renewable at annual intervals. A patient so detained may be discharged by the responsible clinician (formerly known as the responsible medical officer (RMO)).

At any time the patient or, within certain limitations, his or her nearest relative may also make application to a Mental Health Tribunal (MHT), at regular intervals. Under section 117(2) of the MHA 1983 as amended, after-care must be provided for those who cease to be detained under section 37 of that Act and who leave hospital.

The implementation of such after-care is currently the responsibility of the Primary Care Trust (PCT) or Local Health Board (LHB), and of the local social services authority in co-operation with relevant voluntary agencies.

Restriction orders
Section 41 of the 1983 Act (as amended) enables the Crown Court or an appellate court (but *not* a magistrates' court) to make a restriction order. The criteria for making such an order are as follows:

1. That, following conviction, it appears to the court, having regard to:

   (a)   the nature of the offence,

   (b)   the offender's antecedents; and

   (c)   the risk of his or her committing further offences if discharged, that a restriction order is necessary *for the protection of the public from serious harm* [my emphasis].

2. That at least one of the doctors authorised under section 12(2) of the Act whose written evidence is before the court has also given that evidence orally.

The criterion I have italicised above did not appear in the Mental Health Act 1959 and was inserted in the 1983 Act to ensure that only those offender-patients who were considered likely to constitute a serious risk to the public would be subjected to the serious restrictions on liberty that follow the making of such an order (see below). *Serious* harm to the public is not defined in the Act.

Until quite recently, little was known about judges' views and considerations when making a restriction order. However, a study by Quarshi and Shaw (2008) has thrown some light on this matter. Of an admittedly small sample of 12 judges interviewed, there was a unanimous view expressed that 'where a hospital order was being considered involving a serious offence a psychiatrist should take a firm view on whether a restriction order was also required'. Furthermore, the interviewees stated that they would also anticipate a positive recommendation from psychiatrists in cases involving homicide, arson and serious sexual and violent offences. There has been a modest increase in the number of restriction orders made (Quarshi and Shaw, 2008).

A restriction order places serious curbs on the liberty of the offender-patient as follows:

(a) The offender-patient cannot be given leave of absence from the hospital (as he or she can be under non-restricted orders), be transferred elsewhere, or be discharged by the responsible clinician without the consent of the Secretary of State.

(b) The Secretary of State may remove the restrictions if he or she considers they are no longer needed to protect the public from serious harm. Should the order continue in force without the restriction clause, it has the same effect as an order made under section 37 of the Act.

(c) The Secretary of State may, at any time, discharge the offender-patient absolutely or subject to conditions. In considering those restricted cases: (a) which were considered to be particularly problematic; (b) which were considered to be in need of special care in assessment; and (c) where there might have been a fear of possible future risk to the public, the Secretary of State would, in the past, have sought the advice of his or her Advisory Board on Restricted Patients (formerly known as the 'Aarvold Board').[1] The board was stood down in 2003, largely because of the increased power given to tribunals and the development of their expertise in assessment of risk.

Under Section 73 of the 1983 Act (as amended) a Mental Health Tribunal (MHT) may exercise its own powers concerning restricted patients in the following manner:

1. The tribunal *shall* order the patient's *absolute* discharge if it is satisfied that:
    (a) an offender-patient is not now suffering from mental disorder as specified in the Act which

---

1. Named after the late Sir Carl Aarvold, Recorder of London and chairman of the Committee of Inquiry into the Activities of Graham Frederick Young (1947-1990) — 'The Saint Albans Poisoner'.

makes it appropriate for him or her to be detained
in hospital for medical treatment; or

(b) it is not necessary for the health and safety of the
offender-patient or for the protection of other persons
that he or she should receive such treatment; and

(c) it is not appropriate for the offender-patient to remain
liable to be recalled to hospital for further treatment.

In the important legal case of *R v. K* (1990) it was held that
a tribunal which was satisfied that the restricted patient was not
suffering from a mental or psychopathic disorder was nevertheless
entitled to order the conditional discharge of the patient and was
not, as had hitherto been held to be the case, obliged to order his
or her absolute discharge. The court appeared to have in mind the
possibility of a need for a residual power to recall the patient in the
event of a relapse at some future date.

A conditionally discharged offender-patient may be recalled to
hospital by the Secretary of State at any time during the duration of
the restriction order, but the patient has to be referred to a Mental
Health Tribunal for a prompt hearing into the recall, the reasons for
it and any representations the offender-patient may wish to make.
It was also held in 1990 by the Court of Appeal in *ex parte K*[2] that
the Home Secretary did not have to rely on medical evidence in
order to recall a restricted patient to hospital, even if medical opinion was of the view that the patient was not suffering from mental
disorder. This wide discretion was held to lie entirely in the hands
of the Secretary of State, and the public interest would, if necessary,
take precedence. However, this view was subsequently challenged
by the offender-patient who took his case to the European Court
of Human Rights, and won. The court held that, in the absence of
an emergency, there had been a breach of Article 5(1) in recalling

2.   See *R v. Merseyside Mental Health Review tribunal, ex parte K* [1990] 1 All
     ER 694; *R v. Secretary of State for the Home Department, ex parte K* [1990] 3
     All ER 562.

'K' — the appellant — without up-to-date medical evidence that he was suffering from a true mental disorder (*K v. United Kingdom* 1998 BMLT 20). An order for conditional discharge may contain a range of requirements held to be conducive to the welfare of the offender-patient and, more importantly, for the protection of the public.[3]

Hospital and limitation directions

Section 46 of the Crime (Sentences) Act 1997 introduced a new disposal — a hospital direction — which is to be found in sections 45A and 45B of the Mental Health Act 1983 (as amended); it is commonly known in the vernacular as a 'hybrid order'. A hospital direction is defined in the 1983 Act as

> a direction that, instead of being removed to and detained in a
> prison, the offender may be removed to and detained in such hospital
> as may be specified in the direction.

The court may also add a 'limitation direction' which, to all intents and purposes, is similar in effect to a restriction order made under section 41 of the 1983 Act. The disposal is only available to a Crown Court (or on an appeal from that court). Its purpose is to ensure that should a mentally disordered offender not respond to hospital treatment he or she may be transferred to prison.

Transfer of prisoners found to be mentally disordered

Sections 47-52 of the Mental Health Act 1983 (as amended) enable the Secretary of State to order the transfer of sentenced or unconvicted prisoners from prison to hospital if they are found to be suffering from mental disorder as defined in the Act. Under the provisions of section 47, an order in respect of a *sentenced* prisoner *may* be made without restrictions, but it will be much more likely to be made with restrictions under the provisions of section 49. If

---

3.   See previous page.

the Secretary of State is notified by the responsible consultant or a Mental Health Tribunal that such a person no longer needs treatment for mental disorder, there are two possibilities open to him:

1. If the offender-patient has become eligible for parole or has earned statutory remission, he or she can order his or her discharge.

2. Alternatively, he or she can order that the patient be remitted to prison to serve the remainder of his or her sentence. Despite attempts on the part of the government to obviate delays in transferring mentally disordered offenders from prison to hospital, problems continue. One difficulty is that acutely mentally ill prisoners do not always conform to advice to take anti-psychotic medication. Such medication cannot be enforced inside a prison because healthcare arrangements within a prison are not designated as hospital provision for the purposes of the relevant mental health legislation.

'Psychiatric probation orders'

The heading has been placed in quotation marks because although they are commonly known as 'psychiatric probation orders' their correct title under legislation is a mental health treatment requirement (MHTR) under a community order. This type of provision has been available under statute since the Criminal Justice Act of 1948, but is now provided for under the Criminal Justice Act 2003 (see sections 207, 208). This permits such treatment provided:

1. A hospital, or other establishment, will receive him or her and is willing to provide treatment by a registered medical practitioner or chartered psychologist.

2. The court has before it the oral or written evidence of

one doctor (approved under Section 12(2) Mental Health Act 1983 (as amended)) indicating that the offender's condition requires, and may be susceptible to, treatment (but is not such as to warrant his or her detention in pursuance of a hospital or guardianship order). Such an order may be on an in-patient or out-patient basis.

3. As far as a hospital or other institution is concerned, the offender-patient has informal status and there is no power to detain him or her compulsorily (as there is under the provisions of the Mental Health Act). Should the offender-patient leave, the probation officer (case manager) may take action for breach of a requirement of the order. However, it is not open to the court to sanction proceedings for a breach of the order if, for example, the offender-patient refuses a physical form of treatment such as electro-convulsive therapy (ECT). Such orders are of use in cases of milder forms of mental disorder and where it is considered there is no indication of potential serious harm to the offender and/or the public. The limited research that has been carried out into this form of treatment indicates that it is useful in circumstances where there is good co-operation between psychiatric services and the probation service.

Secure Provision

Hospital provision: high security, semi-secure provision and low secure accommodation
A number of mentally disordered offenders will be detained in ordinary psychiatric hospitals. Those who have committed grave crimes, and who are considered to be an immediate danger to the public if at large may, as will be seen shortly, be detained in a high security (formerly known as a 'special') hospital.

In the latter stages of their rehabilitation in the community, such offender-patients may be transferred to an ordinary psychiatric hospital or, more likely, to a medium, and subsequently perhaps, to a low security unit. Until fairly recently, due to the absence of these less secure units and a reluctance on the part of ordinary psychiatric hospitals to take offender-patients, some of them might remain in conditions of high security for far longer than their condition or the safety of the public warranted. The situation is not so serious today, but sadly there are still some instances of lengthy delays in transfer.

Over the years there have been a number of problems in developing the *range* of units required to meet the varied problems presented by all offender-patients:

- *Firstly*, in the past, the secure units tended to be seen as an answer to the problem of the management of the difficult or disruptive patient detained in *ordinary* psychiatric hospitals (It is important to note here that about one third of offender-patients detained in one or other of the three high security hospitals—to be described shortly—are not offenders, but have been transferred to high security accommodation because of their severely disruptive or violent behaviour in other settings). To some extent the situation has been eased in recent years by the establishment of special units catering for such patients who demonstrate what has come to be known as 'challenging behaviour'.

- *Secondly*, secure units have tended to be seen as 'mini-high-security' hospitals.

- *Thirdly*, most of the medium secure units were designed to take offender-patients for a maximum of two years. A number of such patients have longer term needs for some form of secure accommodation. To meet this need, a small number of low-security units have now been set up. They are seen largely as a final 'staging post' before final return to rehabilitation in the open community (for further details see Prins, 2010).

High security (formerly special) hospitals

Under the provisions of section 4 of the National Health Service and Community Care Act 1990, the Secretary of State for Social Services is required to provide and maintain such institutions as are necessary for persons subject to detention under the mental health legislation who, in his or her opinion, require conditions of special security because of their 'dangerous, violent or criminal propensities'. However, as already noted above, about one third of all such detained patients are *not* offenders, but detained because of their difficult, disruptive or violent behaviour in ordinary psychiatric or mental handicap hospitals.

There are three (formerly four) high security hospitals in England, Broadmoor, Rampton and Ashworth (formerly Moss Side and Park Lane) but none in Wales or Northern Ireland. The State Hospital at Carstairs in Scotland is the approximate equivalent of an English high security hospital and the Central Hospital at Dundrum in Dublin performs in the Republic of Ireland some of the functions of its UK counterparts. Because Northern Ireland has no high security hospital it sends a few of its more dangerous offender-patients to Carstairs or, more frequently, to Ashworth.

The former 'special hospitals' have had a long and, from time to time, somewhat chequered history. Formerly administered directly by the Department of Health, subsequently by a specially created health authority — the Special Hospitals Service Authority (SHSA) — they have now been merged with general NHS provision. The aim is to bring these establishments alongside more general psychiatric practice and to reduce the isolation that seems to have plagued them over the years.

The secure hospitals themselves

In more detail the high security hospitals are:

- *Broadmoor* in Berkshire is the oldest of the hospitals having been established in 1863. Once beset by severe overcrowding, some relief was afforded by the building of Park Lane Hospital (now Ashworth Complex, below). However, the provision for female patients has been the subject of continued criticism in recent years and, at one time, its handling of ethnic minority (particularly African-Caribbean) patients left something to be desired.

- *Rampton* in North Nottinghamshire was established in 1914 and in its earlier days tended to specialise in the management of mentally impaired offender-patients. It now has a more mixed population and there has been a concentration on work with the severely personality disordered, notably those considered to be dangerous (see earlier discussion of DSPD patients in *Chapter 3*). Overcrowding was once a serious problem, and the hospital was the subject of an intensive inquiry into allegations of ill-treatment of patients. However, in the last three decades or so, the hospital has shaken off its 'backwater' status and been revitalised by the introduction of more pro-active review processes and more forward-looking staff at all levels.

- *Ashworth Complex* is located at Maghull, Liverpool. The complex consists of the former Moss Side (established 1933) and Park Lane (established 1974) hospitals. At one time, Moss Side took mainly mentally impaired patients, but following integration with Park Lane, it now takes all three categories — the learning disabled, the mentally ill and the severely anti-social personality disordered.

The high security hospitals have come in for a good deal of criticism in the past, some of it justified. However, even their severest critics acknowledge that such institutions have to undertake a tremendously difficult task in attempting to combine containment, clinical treatment and rehabilitation in a climate of opinion that does not give high priority to the care of the 'mad and the bad'. There have been abuses, as witnessed in the highly critical report of the inquiry into conditions at Ashworth (Department of Health, 1992), and a further inquiry into managerial and other deficiencies at the personality disorder unit at the same hospital (Fallon *et al*, 1992).

In the past there have been calls for the high security hospitals to be closed down and be replaced by smaller units. Professional opinion would seem to suggest that the expertise that *does* reside in the secure hospitals needs to be maintained and not dissipated.

Provision for Scotland and Northern Ireland

The clientele of the State Hospital at Carstairs in Scotland (established in 1944) are, to all intents and purposes, much the same as those in the high secure hospitals south of the border. Carstairs normally houses some 200 or so offender-patients, the majority suffering from psychotic illness. As already indicated, it very occasionally receives patients from Northern Ireland.

The Republic of Ireland (Eire)

The Central Hospital at Dundrum has a predominantly male population of some 100 or so offender-patients, about half of whom are said to suffer from schizophrenic illness. A large percentage of these patients are the subjects of transfer from prison.

Penal Provisions

Prison psychiatric services

Eighteenth century legislation required prisons to appoint a physician, and an organized full-time medical service began with the establishment of the Prison Commission in 1887. Such appointments can be seen as the forerunners of a range of other professional appointments which were subsequently to swell the ranks of prison staffs, for example chaplains, psychologists, specialist nursing officers, probation officers (formerly prison welfare officers), education personnel and works and occupations staff.

The history of mental health services in prisons reveals that there were a number of early attempts to describe and classify mentally disordered offenders received into prison. It is possibly not widely known that, over the years, prison medical staff have also had general oversight of the total care of *both prisoners and prison staff and also a concern with environmental health matters.*

Such work has now become a National Health Service (NHS) responsibility and the specific post of prison medical officer is being phased out. Sadly, as stated earlier, there are still a number of mentally disordered offenders who should be in hospital (though the number of 'transfer directions' under the Mental Health Act has increased modestly in recent years), and an even greater number who, whilst not fulfilling the strict criteria for transfer under the mental health legislation, would benefit from better psychiatric oversight and management.

Three other developments should be noted.

- *Firstly,* the report entitled *The Future Organisation of Prison Health Care* published in 1999 set out the policy of prison health care being provided by a partnership with the NHS based upon the principle of equivalence.

- *Secondly*, prison 'mental health in-reach services' which have seen a process of rapid development.

- *Thirdly*, in 2001 the Department of Health, HM Prison Service and the National Assembly for Wales published an important document setting out a strategy for the development and modernising of mental health services in prisons (Department of Health, 2001).

Supervision in the Community

At some point in their careers, attempts will be made to re-locate offender-patients within the community. Those dealt with through the penal system, even though they may have mental health problems, will be dealt with through release on parole, or life licence. Those who have been dealt with under the terms of a hospital order with restrictions will be released on what is known as a 'conditional discharge'. Supervision of those dealt with through the penal system will be undertaken by a probation officer (now also called case managers) and, if there are mental health problems, supervision may also include psychiatric intervention.

Those released through the mental health system will be supervised by either a probation officer or a local authority social worker.[4] At one time, the supervision of restricted patients was almost always undertaken by the probation service; today, supervision is more likely to be undertaken by a local authority social worker. Individual circumstances will govern the choice. If the offender-patient has been previously well-known to the probation service, then it will most likely be the probation service who will be asked to supervise. If additional community resources are required, such as a hostel or

4.   There are plans under which community supervision may be passed to the private or voluntary sector although it is not clear that this would extend to such expert and sensitive areas of probation work (or social work) as mental health arrangements.

day-care facility, then social services will be most likely to be chosen.

In addition to social supervision, almost without exception, the offender-patient will also be under the care and supervision of a named psychiatrist and perhaps a community psychiatric nurse. In both penal and health care orders for release there will be specific requirements, such as:

- place of residence,
- notification of change of address, etc.; and
- any other requirements that are deemed to be in the interests of the offender/offender-patient and, *importantly, the safety of the public.*

Issues relating to public safety and the assessment and management of risk are extremely important. For a comprehensive discussion of the issues involved in the assessment of risk, see the large-scale compilation of papers in Nash and Williams (2010). In restricted cases, it is essential that there is open and constructive liaison between the social supervisor and the psychiatrist. Clear procedures for this should be established between the parties involved — offender-patient — social supervisor — psychiatrist and community nurse (This is essential in the case of the psychopathic offender-patient).

The Ministry of Justice (formerly the Home Office) issues guidelines on best practice and these are up-dated from time-to-time. Not infrequently, decisions have to be made at a time of crisis. For example, an offender-patient's behaviour may have deteriorated to the extent that recall to hospital may need to be considered or, in the case of a parolee or life licensee, recall to prison. The worker carrying responsibility for the case (and by definition this will almost always be a complex and difficult one) should have easy access to their line management for support and advice. Access for further advice from the relevant department of the Ministry of Justice (Mental Health Unit or Parole Unit) is essential.

Cases in which advice would need to be sought would include those where:

- there appears to be an actual or potential risk to the public;
- contact with the offender/offender-patient has been lost;
- there has been a substantial breach of the discharge conditions; or
- the individual's behaviour suggests a need for recall for further in-patient treatment; or
- he or she has been charged with, or convicted of, a further offence.

An offender-patient who is recalled to hospital by order of the Secretary of State has to have his or her case referred to a Mental Health Tribunal[5] within one month of his or her recall. In deciding whether or not to issue a warrant for recall, the Secretary of State will treat each case on its merits. If an offender-patient has been hospitalised in the past for very serious violence or homicide, even comparatively minor irregularities of conduct or failure to co-operate within the terms of the conditional discharge *might* well be sufficient to merit the consideration of recall.

Similar considerations apply in relation to offenders released on parole or life licence. If all goes well, the conditions of a life licence, such as the requirement to live in a specific place, to report to a probation officer, to receive visits or not to take specific employments, may be cancelled — but customarily not before at least four or five years have elapsed; the life licence itself remains in force for life.

As noted earlier, in the case of conditionally discharged restricted patients, the requirements for supervision, or the order for conditional discharge itself, may be lifted by the Secretary of State or by an MHT.

---

5.   Formerly known as MHRTs: see Footnote 7 in *Chapter 3*.

Other National Decision-making and Advisory Bodies

Brief reference has been made to the mechanism of parole, to the Mental Health Tribunal and to the Home Secretary's one-time Advisory Board on Restricted Patients. Each of these is now considered in slightly more detail.

The Parole Board

The arrangements for release on parole and life licence were introduced in the Criminal Justice Act of 1967 and became operational in 1968. They have been amended in major fashion from time to time. The Act of 1967 established the board as an independent body, appointed by the Home Secretary, to offer him or her advice and to take decisions on his or her behalf on the early release of determinate or life-sentence prisoners. More recent enactments and rulings have increased the categories of prisoners who are made subject to parole supervision.

Over the years the independence of the Parole Board has been further marked, for example, by its establishment as an Executive Non-Departmental Public Body in 1996. In its mission statement the board is described as:

> An independent body that works with others to protect the public by risk assessment of prisoners in order to decide whether they can be safely released into the community.
>
> Parole Board, Annual Report, 2012.

Concern has been expressed as to the *real* extent of the board's independent status. This independence has been the subject of review in the Queen's Bench Division of the High Court's Administrative Court.

That court found that although 'there is no question about the independence of mind and impartiality of members of the board' and 'no sign of any attempt by the executive to influence individual cases' there is a valid basis for concern regarding the board's independence. The court in its judgment went on to declare 'that the present arrangements for the Parole Board do not sufficiently demonstrate its objective independence of the Secretary of State as required by English Common Law and [the European Convention on Human Rights] Article 5(4)', as reported by Stone (2008).[6]

The work of the board has been accompanied by a considerable increase in the size of its membership. Under the terms of the 1967 Act, it was required to include amongst its members the following categories of persons:

- a person who holds, or has held, judicial office
- a psychiatrist
- a person who has experience of the supervision or after-care of discharged prisoners (usually a chief or assistant chief probation officer); and
- a person who has made a study of the causes of crime and the treatment of offenders (usually an academic criminologist).

The board currently includes a number of members of each of these categories; in addition, it now includes forensic and clinical psychologists and its 'independent' members are qualified by a range of varied experiences to make significant contributions to the board's work. Current membership of the board consists of a full-time chairman, deputy chairman, two full-time members, and some 250 or so other members (These are listed in detail at p 85 *et seq* in the board's Annual Report, 2012).

---

6.   Article 5 deals with the right to liberty and security. Article 5(4) states: 'Everyone who is deprived of his liberty by arrest or detention shall be entitled to take proceedings by which the lawfulness of his detention shall be decided speedily by a court and his release ordered if the detention is not lawful'. The reference is to Stone N (2008) 'Independence of the Parole Board,etc.': see the *Select Bibliography* at the end of this work.

The vast increase in membership has in part been occasioned by the increase in the prison population and the various categories of prisoners receiving oral hearings. The management of the board's practice has involved a variety of sub-committees dealing with various aspects of the board's work.

The selection process for members has become more intensive. When I served on the board in the late-1970s and early-1980s, not only were numbers much smaller (some 40 plus as I recall), but the 'selection' process was much less formal. One day I received a personal letter from the then Home Secretary (Merlyn Rees) asking if I would accept appointment to the board in the category of criminologist. No formal interview. I was invited to have lunch with the then chairman of the board, Sir Louis Petch and the then secretary, Henry Gonsalves at Sir Louis' club. There was little in the way of formal training as there is today.

Members used to be appointed for a three-year term, renewable for a further period. This has now been changed to five years renewable for a further period of five years (subject to successful performance) with a maximum of ten years.

The complexities of the board's operations and management may be seen in the board's latest Annual Report which runs to one hundred pages. Readers wishing to obtain further details of these matters should consult that report, which can be downloaded at www.official-documents.gov.uk and from the board's website at www.justice.gov.uk (hard copies are not currently available).

The Mental Health Review Tribunal (MHRT)

As noted in *Chapter 3*, Mental Health Review Tribunals (as they were then called)[7] were introduced by the Mental Health Act 1959. They were intended to serve as a replacement for the role of the lay magistracy under previous lunacy legislation in safeguarding the rights of patients subject to detention; they also replaced some of

_____

7.   See Footnote 5 to this chapter..

the functions of an earlier body, the Board of Control, to which a patient could make representations against detention in hospital.

As noted earlier, the role and scope of the tribunals were extended under the Mental Health Act 1983; which gave greater opportunities for appeal against detention and for the automatic review of patients' cases at regular intervals if they had not applied for this themselves. The MHRT is a *judicial* body and has considerable statutory powers which are independent of any government agency such as the Ministry of Justice or Department of Health.

The main purpose of the tribunal is to review the cases of compulsorily detained patients and, if the relevant criteria are satisfied, to direct their discharge. This task involves examination of complex and often conflicting elements giving rise to concern for the liberty of the patient (or offender-patient) on the one hand and, as with the Parole Board, the protection of the public on the other.

Panels normally consist of three members:

- a legal member who chairs the panel,;
- a medical member (almost always a psychiatrist of considerable experience); and
- a so-called 'lay' member, who is neither a lawyer nor a doctor.

All three tribunal members have equal status, and an equal role in the decision-making process and in drafting the reasons for the final decision. Hearings are almost always in private but, in rare circumstances, a patient may request a public hearing. These days patients are almost always legally represented. In particularly difficult or possibly contentious cases, and other interested parties, such as the Ministry of Justice, may be legally represented, usually by counsel.

Tribunals have not been without their critics (See Peay, 1989). Two inquiries into homicides committed by former offender-patients also made for serious criticisms of the system.

In the first of these, the case of Andrew Robinson, details of his original offence were inadequate so that the tribunal had to make decisions on imperfect evidence. At one of his tribunals, the patient had refused to be examined by the medical member (a requirement under the Tribunal Rules). Despite this, the tribunal went ahead, determined the case and gave the patient an absolute discharge. The inquiry team acknowledged that at the various tribunal hearings the members were often having to act upon the information before them, and that this information was often seriously inadequate (Blom-Cooper *et al*, 1995).

In the second case, that of Jason Mitchell, the inquiry team made further criticisms of tribunal practice. The first of these concerned the making of a deferred conditional discharge that contained requirements beyond the tribunal's legal remit. Blom-Cooper (1996) and his colleagues made a number of recommendations:

(a)   Clinical psychologists should be added to the list of 'lay' members who can be appointed to MHTs;

(b)   MHTs should have available more detailed information about an offender-patient's index offence (This was subsequently remedied by the Ministry of Justice);

(c)   In restricted cases (as was Mitchell's), the medical member of the tribunal should preferably be a forensic-psychiatrist;

(d)   MHT members should be afforded follow-up; and in those cases where an offender-patient had re-offended in serious fashion after discharge, a confidential retrospective review should be held.

The Home Secretary's Advisory Board on Restricted Patients

Following the conviction and sentence of the late psychopathic offender-patient — Graham Frederick Young (1947-1990) — for murder by poisoning, the then Home Secretary, acting on the recommendation of the subsequent inquiry into Young's case, established a non-statutory advisory committee (known then as the 'Aarvold Board') to advise him in those restricted cases: (a) which were considered to be particularly problematic; (b) which were considered to need special care in assessment; and (c) where there was thought to be a fear of possible future risk to the public. This committee, subsequently known as the Home Secretary's Advisory Board on Restricted Patients, merely proffered advice to the Home Secretary. In more recent times, it had dealt with very few cases and its workload decreased to the extent that, as already noted, it was stood down, in September 2003.

Questions

1. Are the provisions concerning offenders with mental health problems:

   (a) adequate

   (b) safe enough for the protection of the public

   (c) sufficiently balanced for the needs of 'patients'

   (d) capable of improvement.

2. Concerning secure hospitals, after reading this chapter, what do you now understand happens 'behind the walls' of such establishments in the case of psychopaths?

Suggestions for Further Reading

Blom-Cooper, L QC, Hally, H and Murphy, E (1995), *The Falling Shadow: One Patient's Mental Health Care: 1978-1993*. London: Duckworth.

Blom-Cooper, L QC, Grounds, A, Parker, A and Taylor, M (1996) *The Case of Jason Mitchell: Report of the Independent Panel of Inquiry*. London: Duckworth.

Department of Health (1992) *Report of the Committee of Inquiry into Complaints About Ashworth Hospital* (Chairman, Sir Louis Blom-Cooper, QC). Cmnd 2028, I and II. London: HMSO.

Department of Health (1999) *The Future Organization of Prison Health Care*. London: Department of Health.

Prins (2010) *Offenders Deviants or Patients: Explorations in Clinical Criminology* (4th edn.). London: Routledge.

Chapter Five
Concluding Comments

'Behold I will unfold a Mystery'[1]

I Corinthians 15: Verse 51, New English Bible.

'A devil, a born devil, on whose nature nurture
never can stick; on whom my pains, humanely
taken, all, all lost, quite lost'

Shakespeare, Prospero in The Tempest, Act IV, Scene 1.

Both these quotations reflect the problems in understanding psychopathic disorder—a mysterious condition—as I hope to have demonstrated earlier in this book, and one not easily amenable to management, as reflected in Prospero's somewhat despairing comments. This is not to say that *no* progress has been made. If some of my comments in earlier chapters have spurred readers to explore the issues further, then this book will have served its purpose.

Ill or Evil?

Readers will be struck perhaps by the absence thus far of any meaningful discussion of the concept of evil in relation to psychopaths (or others). It seems to me that the subject is best addressed by those well versed in social philosophy and theology. However, I will offer a few observations. In my opinion, it is not a helpful approach to describe individuals as being 'evil'. This said, it is an understandable reaction on the part of those who have suffered at the hands of some of the individuals referred to at various places in this book.

---

1. The words immortalised by George Frideric Handel in *Messiah*. Sometimes expressed as 'Tell you a Mystery', or 'Shew You'. In my view these are more powerful words than those given above and reflect more sharply the context of the quotation.

Indeed, the use of the word 'evil' does little to aid our understanding of psychopathic behaviour. My one modest 'foray' into the debates about the use of the term came about some years ago, in the following way. The then Editor of the *British Journal of Psychiatry* — Professor Greg Wilkinson — invited me to write an editorial on 'Psychiatry and the Concept of Evil' (Prins, 1994). His request was prompted by several contemporary cases of extreme violence and, in particular, the killing of the toddler James Bulger by the ten-year-old boys Robert Thompson and Jon Venables.

The horrific and brutally executed killing shocked the nation. All manner of explanations were proffered for the behaviour of the two perpetrators. Some cast the established church in the role of 'scapegoat' for failing to provide moral guidance; forensic mental health and criminal justice professionals cited the importance of family background and psychopathology linked to possible neurological impairment of some kind.

The police invoked the concept of evil (though, to their credit, for the most part kept a professional distance). A comment attributed to the trial judge suggested that viewing 'video nasties' might have been an influence on the two boys.

Earlier in this book I have quoted a number of mental health authorities who suggest that even very small infants can have murderous feelings; this raises the uncomfortable possibility that even they or other young children may commit 'evil' acts such as homicide. It is important to point out at this stage that, fortunately, such acts are exceedingly rare. One case that attracted a great deal of attention was that of Mary Bell some years earlier. With an accomplice, she killed two small boys. Her story is described sensitively and yet graphically by the late Gita Sereny in her book *Cries Unheard* (1998).

The phenomenon of children who kill in the UK, Europe and elsewhere, its recurring but relatively rare nature and wide range of explanations, was also examined in a collection of accounts by leading medical and psychiatric and other experts under the auspices of the former British Juvenile and Family Courts Society (Cavadino *et al*, 1996), Writing in that work and in relation to the Bulger case, Gita Sereny noted how use of the word 'evil' can often be a societal rather than a professionally considered response:

> 'But did people ask "What made it happen?". Some people did of course, but not enough. They were "evil". If there families were talked about at all, they had done it because they belonged to "them" … the poor, the disadvantaged, the people who drink, the people who do not care for their homes or their children'.

In general, we find it far easier to try to understand such serious acts when committed by adults. However, this is not always the case. I recall the comment by the bewildered and distressed Governor of HM Prison Strangeways after the riots at that establishment when he said 'evil forces have been at work' (As reported in *The Independent*, 9 May, 1990, p 1).

This assumption of innocence in childhood can, perhaps, be explained in part by our need to exclude from our thinking and feeling (denial) the very possibility of the worst 'evil' deeds by adults being carried out by those we so blithely assume to be innocent (i.e. children).

A question often raised is whether 'evil' exists as some external force—'out there' as it were—or whether it can only exist, as George Gifford suggested in the 17th century 'in the hearts of men' (*A Dialogue Concerning Witches and Witchcraft*, 1603). Perhaps its existence as a malign external force is best exemplified in the phenomenon of demonic possession (see Prins, 1990).

Two contrasting views on the phenomenon of evil will, I hope, sharpen our awareness of the problems of where we should locate it and who should deal with it. The first is from a lecture to medical students by one of psychiatry's founding fathers, Henry Maudsley, in the late-19th century. He said:

'Medical science of the future will have a great deal to say ... respecting the highest concerns of man's nature and conduct of his life (and) ... will enter a domain which has hitherto been given up exclusively to the moral philosopher and the preacher'.

Quoted in Wootton, 1980, p 525.

We can now contrast this somewhat grandiose claim with a more modest one by an experienced circuit judge—His Honour Judge Geoffrey Jones. The editor of the journal and I had asked him to provide a brief commentary on my editorial. He wrote:

'My own present, unresolved thoughts are that "evil" is within the realm of theologians and moral philosophers. Doctors, judges and lawyers would do well to concern themselves with bad deeds and bad health, that is deeds, which society has determined as criminal. If the perpetrators of bad deeds are not sick, they should be punished according to law. If they are sick, they should be treated'.

Jones, 1994: 302.[2]

An Eye to the Future

Readers may consider this is a more modest aspiration than Maudsley's. From my point of view the only problem with Judge Jones' statement is, to use old fashioned words, that of determining the borderline area between 'sickness' and 'sin'.

So, what are the main problems for the future in relation to understanding and managing those designated as psychopathically disordered?

---

2. The areas for debate as exemplified in the two quotations above are well illustrated in a module on 'The Psychology of Evil' delivered by my colleague Dr Sarah Hodgkinson of our department at Leicester University. The popularity of the module is evidenced by the fact that it is invariably over-subscribed.

- *First*, as suggested in *Chapter 2*, there have been advances in understanding those aspects of brain functioning that may be responsible for the types of behaviour we designate as psychopathic.

- *Second*, to achieve a better understanding of developmental child psychology and the role of parents and other close caring figures.

- *Third*, attempts to further our understanding of the influence of genetic factors and the complex web of relationships between these and social/familial influences. This area of endeavour owes much to the detailed explorations by Sir Michael Rutter and his co-workers referred to earlier in this book.

- *Fourth*, attempts to further our understanding of the impact of available forms of therapeutic endeavour and the extent to which forms of therapy work best for different manifestations of psychopathic behaviour. It is unfortunate that, at times, polarisation occurs between the various proponents of therapy — for example those using applied psychoanalytic psychotherapy and those espousing behavioural techniques. This attitude is wasteful of effort and counter-productive.

- *Fifth*, we need the results of long-term outcome studies into the benefits of management/treatment for dangerous and severe personality disorder (see the discussion in *Chapter 3*).

- *Sixth*, a more critical appraisal of the various rating and allied scales in use for predicting and managing psychopathic behaviour. Occasionally these have been espoused somewhat uncritically. It is worth recalling that a foremost authority in the field, Professor Robert Hare, has urged caution in accepting uncritically his work on developing the Psychopathy Check List (now the PCL-R). In the UK, the work of Professor Anthony Maden (2007) has also been important. My own 'take' on reading his work on risk assessment in forensic mental health is that assessment scales of one kind or another can give useful insights into the extent to which individuals as a group *may* behave in the future, so that one can be made conscious of the possibility of serious violent behaviour. However, this insight by no means precludes a careful appraisal of an *individual* in a range of possible precipitating circumstances.

- *Seventh*, the vital need to endeavour to be aware of one's own demons. Let Banquo in *Macbeth* have the last word. Addressing his fellows just after the discovery of King Duncan's murder he says:

And when we have our naked frailties hid
That suffer in exposure, let us meet
And question this most bloody piece of work
To know it further.

Shakespeare, *Macbeth*, Act II, Scene 3.

Question

I make seven areas for further work.

Can you suggest others?

Select Bibliography

Aigebusi, A. and Tuck, G. (2008) 'Caring Amid Victims and Perpetrators: Trauma and Forensic Mental Health Nursing'. In J. Gordon and G. Kirtchuk (eds) *Psychic Assaults and Frightened Clinicians*. London: Karnac.

Ainsworth, M.D.S. (1962) *The Effects of Maternal Deprivation: A Review of Findings and Controversy in the Context of Research Strategy*. World Health Organization Public Health Papers, No. 14. Geneva: World Health Organization.

Allport, G.W. (1937) *Personality: A Psychological Interpretation*. New York: Holt.

American Psychiatric Association (1994) *Diagnostic and Statistical Manual of Mental Disorders* (4ᵗʰ ed). Washington DC.

Anderson, A.E. (1958) Foreword to *Psychopathic Personalities*. Schneider, K. (Tr. M.W. Hamilton). London: Cassell.

Arnold, C. (2008) *Bedlam: London and its Mad*. London: Simon and Schuster.

Barett, B., Byford, S., Sieveright, H., Cooper, S., Duggan, C. and Tyrer, P. (2009). 'The Assessment of DSPD: Service Use, Cost and Consequences'. *Journal of Forensic Psychiatry and Psychology*, 20: 120-131.

Baron-Cohen, S. (2011) *Zero Degrees of Empathy: A New Theory of Human Cruelty*. London: Allen Lane.

Bavidge, N.M. (1989) *Mad or Bad?* Bristol: Classical Press.

Beck, U. (1998) 'Politics of Risk Society', in J. Franklin (ed.) *The Politics of Risk Society* (pp. 9-22). Cambridge: Polity Press.

Berrios, G.E. (1993) Personality Disorders: A Conceptual History. In: P. Tyrer and G. Stein (eds). *Personality Disorder Reviewed*. London: Gaskell Books.

Blackburn. R. (2007) 'Other Theoretical Models of Psychopathy'. In C.J. Patrick (ed.) *Handbook of Psychopathy*. New York:

Guilford Press.

Blair, J. and Frith, U. (2000) 'Neurocognitive Explanations of Anti-social Personality Disorders'. In *Criminal Behaviour and Mental Health* (Supplement) 10: 566-581.

Blair, J., Mitchell, D. and Blair, K. (2005) *The Psychopath: Emotion and The Brain*. Oxford: Blackwell Publishing.

Blom-Cooper, L. QC, Grounds, A., Parker, A. and Taylor, M. (1996) *The Case of Jason Mitchell: Report of the Independent Panel of Inquiry*. London: Duckworth.

Blom-Cooper, L. QC, Hally, H. and Murphy, E. (1995) *The Falling Shadow: One Patient's Mental Health Care: 1978-1993*. London: Duckworth.

Board, B.J. and Fritzon, K. (2005) Disordered Personalities at Work. *Psychology, Crime and Law*. 11: 17-32.

Bowers, L. (2002) *Dangerous Severe Personality Disorders: Response and Role of the Psychiatric Team*. London: Routledge.

Bowers, L., Carr-Walker, P., Paton, J., Nijman, H.M., Callaghan, P., Allan, T. and Alexander, J. (2005) 'Changes in Attitude to Personality Disorder on a DSPD Unit'. In *Criminal Behaviour and Mental Health*, 15: 171-183.

Bowlby, J. (1946) *Forty-Four Juvenile Thieves: Their Characters and Home Life*. London: Baillière, Tindall and Cox.
(1979) *The Making and Breaking of Affectional Bonds*. London: Tavistock.

Burn, M. (1956) *Mr. Lyward's Answer*. London: Hamish Hamilton.

Burns, T., Yiend, J., Fahy, T., Fitzpatrick, R., Rogers, R., Fazel, S. and Sinclair, J. (2011). 'Treatments for Dangerous Severe Personality Disorder (DSPD)'. In *Journal of Forensic Psychiatry and Psychology*, 22: 411-426.

Burt, C. (1944) *The Young Delinquent* (4th edn.). London: University of London Press.

Callender, J. S. (2010) *Freewill and Responsibility. A Guide For Practitioners*. Oxford: Oxford University Press.

Campling, P. (1996) 'Maintaining the Therapeutic Alliance With Personality Disordered Patients'. In *Journal of Forensic Psychiatry*, 7: 535-550.

Camporesi, P. (1989) *Bread of Dreams: Food and Fantasy in Early Modern Europe*. Cambridge: Polity Press.

Cavadino P, et al (1996) *Children Who Kill*. Hook: Waterside Press.

Chiesa, M. and Fonagy, P. (2003) 'Psychological Treatment of Severe Personality Disorder: A 36-Month Follow Up'. In *British Journal of Psychiatry*, 183: 356-362.

Clarke, B. (1975) *Mental Disorder in Earlier Britain: Exploratory Studies*. Cardiff: University of Wales.

Cleckley, H. (1976) *The Mask of Sanity*. (5th edn.) St. Louis: C. V. Mosby.

Cohen, S. (2002) *Folk Devils and Moral Panics*. (3rd edn.) London: Routledge.

Coid, J. (1993) Current Concepts and Classification in Psychopathic Disorder. In P. Tyrer and G. Stein (eds.). *Personality Disorder Reviewed*. London: Gaskell Books.

Cooke, D.J., Michie, C. and Hart, S.D. (2007) 'Facets of Clinical Psychopathy: Towards Greater Measurement'. In C.J.Patrick (ed) *Handbook of Psychopathy*. New York: Guilford Press.

Cope, R. (1993) 'A Survey of Forensic Psychiatrists' Views on Psychopathic Disorder'. *Journal of Forensic Psychiatry*, 3: 214-235.

Coughlin, L. (2003) 'The Effects of Relocation of Staff Changes on Individuals With a Personality Disorder. *British Journal of Forensic Practice*, 5: 12-17.

Damasio, A.R. (1994) *Descartes Error: Emotion, Rationality and The Human Brain*. New York: Putnam.

Deeley, Q., Daly, E., Surgoladze, S., Tunstall *et al*. (2006) 'Facial Emotion Processing in Criminal Psychopathy: Preliminary Functional Magnetic Resonance Imaging Study'. In *British Journal of Psychiatry* 189: 533-539.

Department of Health (1992) *Report of the Committee of Inquiry into Complaints About Ashworth Hospital* (Chairman Sir Louis Blom-Cooper QC). Cmnd 2028, I and II. London: HMSO.

(1999) *The Future Organisation of Prison Health Care*. London: Department of Health.

(1999) *Report of the Expert Committee: Review of the Mental Health Act, 1983*. (Richardson Committee). London: TSO.

(2003) *Personality Disorder: No Longer a Diagnosis of Exclusion*. London: Department of Health.

Department of Health and Home Office (1994) *Report of the Department of Health and Home Office Working Group on Psychopathic Disorder*. (Chairman Dr. John Reed, CB). London: Department of Health.

Department of Health, HM Prison Service, National Assembly for Wales (2001) *Changing the Outlook. A Strategy For the Development and Modernising of Mental Health Services in Prisons*. London: Department of Health.

Duggan, C. (2007) 'To Move or Not to Move—That is the Question: Some Reflections on the Transfer of DSPD Patients in the Face of Uncertainty'. In *Psychology, Crime and Law*, 13: 113-121.

Esquirol, E. (1838) *Des Maladies Mentales*. (2 Vols.) Paris: Ballière.

Fallon, P. QC, Bluglass, R., Edwards, B. and Daniels, G. (1999) *Report of the Committee of Inquiry into the Personality Disorder Unit, Ashworth Special Hospital*. (2 Vols.). CM4194 (I) and CM4195 (II). London: TSO.

Farrington, D.P. (2007) 'Family Background and Psychopathy.' In Patrick, C.J. (ed.) *Handbook of Psychopathy*. New York: Guilford Press.

Faulks, S. (2007) *Engleby*. London: Hutchinson.

Fennell, P. (2007) *Mental Health: The New Law*. Bristol: Jordan Publishing.

Feracutti, S. (1996) 'Cesare Lombroso (1835-1907)'. In *Journal of Forensic Psychiatry* 7: 130-149.

Ferrito, M., Vetere, A., Adshead, G. and Moore, E. (2012) 'Life

After Homicide: Accounts of Recovery and Redemption of Offender-Patients in a High Security Hospital—A Qualitative Study'. In *Journal of Forensic Psychiatry and Psychology*, 23: 327:344.

Forshaw, D. and Rollin, H. (1990) 'The Development of Forensic Psychiatry in England'. In R. Bluglass and P. Bowden (eds.) *Principles and Practice of Forensic Psychiatry*, pp 61-101. London: Churchill Livingstone.

Fowles, D.C. and Dindo, L. (2007) 'A Dual-Deficit Model of Psychopathy'. In C.J. Patrick (ed.), *Handbook of Psychopathy*. New York: Guilford Press.

Francis, R. QC. (2007). 'The Michael Stone Inquiry: A Reflection'. In *Journal of Mental Health Law*, 15: 41-49.

Gifford, G. (1603), A Dialogue Concerning Witches and Wichcraft. London: The Percy Society (reprint).

Gledhill, K. (2009). 'The First Flight of the Fledgling: The Upper Chamber Tribunal's Substantive Debut'. *Journal of Mental Health Law*, 18: 81-93.

Glueck, B. (1918) 'A Study of 608 Admissions to Sing Sing Prison'. In *Mental Hygiene* 11: 85-151.

Glueck, S. and Glueck, E. (1962) *Family Environment and Delinquency*. London: Routledge and Kegan Paul.

Gordon, J. and Kirtchuk, G. (2008) (eds.). *Psychic Assaults and Frightened Clinicians*. London: Karnac.

Gordon, J., Harding, S., Miller, C. and Xenitidis, K. (2008) 'X-treme Group Analysis: On the Countertransference Edge in In-Patient Work with Forensic Patients'. In Gordon, J. and Kirtchuk, G. *Psychic Assaults and Frightened Clinicians*. London: Karnac.

Greenall, P.V. (2009) 'Assessing High Risk Offenders With Personality Disorders'. In *British Journal of Forensic Practice*, 13: 14-18.

Grieg, D. (2002) *Neither Mad Nor Bad: The Competing Discourses of Psychiatry, Law and Politics*. London: Jessica Kingsley.

Grounds, A. (2001) 'Reforming the Mental Health Act'. *British Journal of Psychiatry*, 179: 387-389.

Gunn J. (1977) *Epileptics in Prison*. London: Academic Press.

(1999) 'The Ashenputtel Principle'. In *Criminal Behaviour and Mental Health*, 10: 73-76.

(2003) 'Psychopathy: An Elusive Concept with Moral Overtones'. In T. Millon, E. Simondson, M. Birkett-Smith and D.R. David (eds.) *Psychopathy: Anti-Social Crime and Violent Behaviour*. New York: Guilford Press.

Haddock, A., Snowden, P., Bolan, M., Parker, J. and Rees, H. (2001) 'Managing Dangerous People With Severe Personality Disorder'. *Psychiatric Bulletin*, 25: 293-296.

Hare, R.D. (1993) *Without Conscience: The Disturbing World of The Psychopath*. New York: Pocket Books.

Hare, R.D., Harpur, T.J., Hakstian, A.R., Forth, A.E., Hart, S.D. and Newman, J.P. (1990) 'The Revised Psychopathy Checklist: Reliability and Factor Structure'. In *Psychiatric Assessment* 2: 338-341.

Hare R.D. (1991) Psychopathy Checklist-Revised. Toronto: Multi-Health Systems.

Hatcher, J. (2008) *The Black Death: An Intimate History*. London: Weidenfeld and Nicolson.

Henderson, D. (1939) *Psychopathic States*. New York: Norton.

Henson, T. and Riordan, S. (2012) 'MAPPA and Detained Patients: Views From Professionals about Referral'. In *Journal of Forensic Psychiatry and Psychology*, 23: 421-434.

Hodgkinson, S. and Prins H. (2011) 'Homicide Law Reform: Coke v. Bumble — Revisited and Re-assessed'. In *Medicine, Science and the Law* 51: 195-202.

Home Office (1939) *Report on the Psychological Treatment of Crime: The East/Hubert Report*. London: HMSO.

Home Office and Department of Health (1999) *People With Severe Personality Disorder: Proposals For Policy Development*. London: Home Office.

Home Office and DHSS (1975) *Report of the Committee on Mentally Abnormal Offenders.* (Butler Committee). Cmnd. 6344. London: HMSO.

House of Commons Estimates Committee (Session 1967-68) (1968) *The Special Hospitals.* London: HMSO.

Howard, J. (1777) *The State of the Prisons in England and Wales and an Account of some Foreign Prisons and Hospitals.* London: Patterson Smith.

Jones, G. (1994) 'Comment on Prins: Psychiatry and the Concept of Evil'. In *British Journal of Psychiatry,* 165: 301-302.

Jones, K. (1993) *Asylums and After: A Revised History of the Mental Health Services: From the Early 18th Century to the Nineteen Hundreds.* London: Athlone Press.

Kendler, K.S., and First, M.B. (2010) 'Alternative Futures For the DSM Revision Process: Iteration v. Paradigm Shift', In *British Journal of Psychiatry* 197: 263-265.

Klawans, H.L. (1990) *Newton's Madness. Further Tales of Clinical Neurology.* London: Bodley Head.

Knop, J., Goodwin, D.W., Jensen, P., Penick, E.C., Pollock, V., Gabrielli, W., Teasdale, T.W. and Mednick, S.A. (1993) 'A 30-Year Follow-Up Study of Sons of Alcholic Men'. In *Acta, Psychiatrica Scandinavica* 75: (Supplement 37) 48-53.

Koch, J.L.A. (1890) *Brief Pointers in Psychiatry: Psychopathic Inferiorities.* (2nd ed). Ravenburg: Maier.

Langton, C. (2007) 'Assessment Implications of "What Works" Research For Dangerous and Severe Personality Disorder (DSPD): Service Evaluation'. *Psychology, Crime and Law,* 13: 97-111.

Lee, T., McLean, D., Moran, P., Jones, H. and Kumar, A. (2008) 'A Pilot Personality Disorder Outreach Service: Development, Findings and Lessons Learnt'. In *Psychiatric Bulletin,* 32: 127-130.

Lodge-Patch, I. (1990) 'Homelessness and Vagrancy', in R. Bluglass and P. Bowden (eds.) *Principles and Practice of Forensic*

Psychiatry, pp 459-466. London: Churchill Livingstone.

Lombroso, C. (1896/7) *Luomo Delinquente* (5ᵗʰ edn.). Torino: Bocca.

Lykken, D .T. (2007) 'Psychopathic Personality: The Scope of the Problem'. In: C.J. Patrick (ed.), *Handbook of Psychopathy*. New York: Guilford Press. (Ch. 1).

Lyman, D.R., and Derefinko, K.J. (2007) 'Psychopathy and Personality'. In C.J. Patrick, (ed), *Handbook of Psychopathy*. New York: Guilford Press. (Ch. 7).

Maden, A. (2011) *Treating Violence: A Guide to Risk Management in Mental Health*. Oxford: Oxford University Press.

Maier, G.J. (1990) 'Psychopathic Disorders: Beyond Counter-Transference'. In *Current Opinion in Psychiatry*, 3: 766-769.

Mark, V.R. and Irvin, F.R. (1970) *Violence and the Brain*. New York: Harper and Row.

Masters, B. (1990) *Gary*. London: Jonathan Cape.

McCord, W. (1982) *The Psychopath and Milieu Therapy: A Longitudinal Study*. New York: Academic Press.

McCord. W. and McCord, J. (1956) *Psychopathy and Delinquency*. Grune and Stratton: London and New York.

McCulloch, J.W. and Prins H. (1978) *Signs of Stress: The Social Problems of Psychiatric Illness*. London: Woburn Press.

McGuffin, P. and Tharpar. A. (2003) 'Genetics and Anti-Social Personality Disorder'. In T. Millon, M. Birkett-Smith and R.D. David, (eds.), *Psychopathy, Anti-Social and Violent Behaviour*. New York: Guilford Press.

Minzberg, M.J. and Siever, L.J. (2007) 'Neuro-chemistry and Pharmacology of Psychopathy and Related Disorders'. In: C.J.Patrick (ed.), *Handbook of Psychopathy*. New York: Guilford Press. (Ch.13).

Morris, T. and Blom-Cooper, L. Q.C. (2011) *Fine Lines and Distinctions: Murder, Manslaughter and the Unlawful Taking of Human Life*. Hook: Waterside Press.

Moss, K. (2009) *Security and Liberty: Restriction by Stealth*.

Basingstoke: Palgrave Macmillan.

(2011) *Balancing Liberty and Security: Human Rights, Human Wrongs*. Basingstoke: Palgrave Macmillan.

Moss, K. and Prins, H. (2006) 'Severe (Psychopathic) Disorder: A Review'. In *Medicine, Science and the Law* 46: 190-207.

Murphy, D. (2007) 'Hare Psychopathy Checklist Revised Profiles of Male Patients With Asperger's Syndrome Detained in High Security Care'. In *Journal of Forensic Psychiatry and Psychology* 18: 120-126.

Nash, M. and Williams, A. (eds) (2010) *Handbook of Public Protection*. Abingdon: Willan/Routledge.

NIHME (2003) *Personality Disorder: No Longer A Diagnosis of Exclusion*. Leeds: Department of Health.

Parker, E. (1985) 'The Development of Secure Provision'. In L. Gostin (ed.) *Secure Provision: A Review of Special Services For the Mentally Ill and Mentally Handicapped in England and Wales*. London: Tavistock.

Parole Board for England and Wales. Annual Report and Account 2011/12, London: TSO.

Patrick, C.J. (ed.) (2007) *Handbook of Psychopathy*. London: Guilford Press.

Peay, J. (1989) *Tribunals on Trial: A Study in Decision Making Under the Mental Health Act 1983*. Oxford: Clarendon Press.

(2000) 'Reform of the Mental Health Act, 1983: Squandering a Lost Opportunity'. In *Journal of Mental Health Law*, 3: 5-15.

Phull, J. and Bartlett, P. (2012) 'Appropriate Medical Treatment: What's in a Word?' *Medicine, Science and the Law*, 52: 71-74.

Pinel, P. (1809) *Traité Médico-Philsophique sur L'Aliénation Mentale* (2nd ed). Paris: Brosson.

Prichard, J.C. (1835) *Treatise on Insanity*. London: Gilbert and Piper.

Prins, H. (1977) 'I Think They Call Them Psychopaths'. In *Prison Service Journal* 28: 8-12.

(1980) *Offenders Deviants or Patients: An Introduction to the Study of Socio-Forensic Problems*. London: Tavistock.

(1990) *Bizarre Behaviours: Boundaries of Psychiatry.* (Ch. 3). London: Tavistock Routledge.

(1993) 'The People Nobody Owns'. In W. Watson and A. Grounds (eds.) *The Mentally Disordered Offender in an Era of Community Care*. Cambridge: Cambridge University Press.

(1994) *Fire Raising: Its Motivation and Management*. London: Routledge.

(1994) 'Psychiatry and the Concept of Evil — Sick in Heart or Sick in Mind'. In *British Journal of Psychiatry*, 165: 297-302.

(1998) 'Characteristics of Consultant Forensic Psychiatrists: A Modest Survey'. In *Journal of Forensic Psychiatry*, 139: 139-149.

(2001) 'Did Lady Macbeth Have a Mind Diseas'd? (A Medico-Legal Enigma)'. In *Medicine, Science and the Law*. 41: 129-134.

(2007) 'The Michael Stone Inquiry: A Somewhat Different Homicide Report'. In *Journal of Forensic Psychiatry and Psychology*, 18: 411-431.

(2010) 'Dangers by Being Despised Grow Great', in M. Nash and A. Williams (eds.) *Handbook of Public Protection*, pp 15-39 Abingdon: Routledge/Willan.

(2010) *Offenders Deviants or Patients: Explorations in Clinical Criminology* (4th edn.). London: Routledge.

Quarshi, I. and Shaw, J. (2008) 'Sections 37/41 Mental Health Act 1983: A Study of Judges' Practice and Assessment of Risk to the Public'. In *Medicine, Science and the Law*, 48: 57-63.

Raine, A. and Yang, Y. (2007) 'The Neuro-Anatomical Basis of Psychopathy: A Review of Brain Imaging Findings'. In C.J. Patrick (ed), *Handbook of Psychopathy*. New York: Guilford Press. (Ch. 14).

Raine, A., Lee, L., Yang, Y. and Colletti, P. (2010). 'Neurodevelopmental Marker For Limbic Maldevelopment in Anti-Social Personality Disorder and Psychopathy'. In *British Journal of Psychiatry* 197: 186-192.

Roberts, A.D.C. and Coid, J.W. (2007) 'Psychopathy and Offending Behaviour: Findings From the National Survey in England and Wales'. In *Journal of Forensic Psychiatry and Psychology* 18: 23-43.

Robertson, J. and Robertson, J. (1967-72) *Young Children in Brief Separation* (Film Series). London: Tavistock: Institute of Human Relations.

Robins, L. (1966) *Deviant Children Grown Up: A Sociological and Psychiatric Study of Sociopathic Personality*. Baltimore: The Williams and Wilkins Foundation.

Roudinesco, E. (2009) *Our Dark Side: A History of Perversion*. Cambridge: Polity Press.

Royal Commission on the Care and Control of the Feeble Minded. (1908) (Radnor Comission) (Cmnd. 4202). London: HMSO.

Royal Commission on the Law Relating to Mental Illness and Mental Deficiency. (1957) (Percy Commission) (Cmnd. 169). London: HMSO.

Rubin, M. (2005) *The Hollow Crown: A History of Britain in the Late Middle Ages*. London: Allen Lane.

Rutter, M. (2006) *Genes and Behaviour: Nature-Nurture Interplay Explored*. Oxford: Blackwell Publishing.

Schmideberg, M. (1949) 'The Analytic Treatment of Major Criminals: Therapeutic Results and Technical Problems'. In Eissler, K.R. (ed.) *Searchlights on Delinquency: New Psychoanalytic Studies*. London: Imago.

Schneider, K. (1958) *Psychopathic Personalities*. (Tr. M. Hamilton). London: Cassell.

Scott, P.D. (1960) 'The Treatment of Psychopaths'. In *British Medical Journal*, 2: 1641-1646.

(1975) *Has Psychiatry Failed in the Treatment of Offenders?* London: Institute for the Study and Treatment of Delinquency. (ISTD).

Sereny, G. (1998) *Cries Unheard: The Story of Mary Bell.* London: MacMillan.

Seto, M.C. and Quinsey, V.L. (2007) 'Toward The Future: Translating Basic Research into Prevention and Treatment Strategies'. In C.J. Patrick (ed.), *Handbook of Psychopathy.* New York: Guilford Press. (Ch. 30).

Sheldon, K. and Krishnan, G. (2009) 'The Clinical and Risk Characteristics of Patients in a Secure Hospital Based DSPD Unit'. In *British Journal of Forensic Practice*, 11: 19-27.

Sheldon, K. and Tennent, A. (2011) 'Considerations For Working With Personality Disordered Patients'. In *British Journal of Forensic Practice*, 13: 41-53.

Shriver, L. (2005) *We Need to Talk About Kevin.* London: Serpent's Tail

Sizmur, S. and Noutch, T. (2005) 'Dangerous and Severe Personality Services'. In *British Journal of Forensic Practice* 7: 33-38.

Slater, E.T.O. (1948) 'Psychopathic Personality as a Genetical Concept'. *Journal of Mental Science* 94: 277-285.

Smartt, U (2001) *Grendon Tales: Stories from a Therapeutic Community.* Hook: Waterside Press.

Snowden, P. and Kane, E. (2003) 'Personality Disorder: No Longer a Diagnosis of Exclusion', *Psychiatric Bulletin* 27: 401-403.

Spence, S., Hunter, A., Farrow, T.F.D., Green, R.D., Leung, D.H., Hughes, C.J. and Ganesan, V. (2004) 'A Cognitive Neuro-Biological Account of Deception: Evidence From Functional Neuro-Imaging'. In *Philosophical Transactions.* Royal Society, London (B) 359: 1755-1762.

Stein, G. (2009) 'Was the Scoundrel (Belial) in the Book of Proverbs a Psychopath?: Psychiatry in the Old Testament'. In *British Journal of Psychiatry* 194: 33.

Stone, N. (2008) 'Independence of the Parole Board'. In *Probation Journal: Journal of Community and Criminal Justice*, 55: 115-116.

Sugarman, P. and Oakley, C. (2012) 'The Evolution of Secure and Forensic Care'. In *Journal of Forensic Psychiatry and Psychology* 23 (June): 279-284.

Taylor, P. (2012) 'Severe Personality Disorder in the Secure Estate—Continuity and Change'. In *Medicine, Science and the Law*, 52: 125-127.

Taylor, R. (2000) *A Seven-Year Reconviction Study of HMP Grendon Therapeutic Community.* Home Office RDS Research Findings, No. 155. London: Home Office.

Tennent, G., Tennent, D., Prins, H. and Bedford, A. (1993) 'Is Psychopathic Disorder a Treatable Condition?' In *Medicine, Science and the Law*, 33: 63-66.

Tiffin, P., Shah, P. and Le Couteur, A. (2007) 'Diagnosing Pervasive Developmental Disorders in a Forensic Mental Health Setting'. In *British Journal of Forensic Practice* 9: 31-40.

Tilt, R., Perry, N. and Martin, C. (2000) *Report of the Review of Security at the High Security Hospitals.* London: Department of Health.

Tilt. R. (2003) Letter, *British Journal of Psychiatry,* 182: 548.

Trebilcock, J. and Weaver, T. (2012) 'Changing Legal Characteristics of DSPD Patients and Prisoners'. In *Journal of Forensic Psychiatry and Psychology*, 23: 237-243.

'It Doesn't Have to be Treatable. MHRT Members' Views About DSPD'. *Journal of Forensic Psychiatry and Psychology,* 23: 244-260.

Trethowan, W. and Sims, A.C.P. (1983) *Psychiatry* (5th edn.), London: Baillière Tindall.

Trevelyan, G.M. (1946) *English Social History: A Survey of Six Centuries—Chaucer-Queen Victoria.* (2nd edn.). London: Longmans Green.

Treves-Brown, C. (1977) 'Who is the Psychopath?' In *Medicine,*

Science and the Law, 17: 56-63.

Tyrer, P. (1990) 'Diagnosing Personality Disorders'. In *Current Developments in Psychiatry* 3: 182-187.

Tyrer, P., Casey, P. and Ferguson, B. (1990) 'Personality Disorders in Perspective'. In *British Journal of Psychiatry* 159: 463-471.

Tyrer, P., Duggan, C., Cooper, S., Crawford, M., Seivewright, H., Rutter, D., Maden, T., Byford, S. and Barett, B. (2010) 'The Success and Failures of the DSPD Experiment: The Assessment and Management of Severe Personality Disorder'. In *Medicine, Science and the Law*, 50: 95-99.

Tyrer, P., Duggan, C. and Coid, J. (2003) 'Ramifications of Personality Disorder in Clinical Practice'. In *British Journal of Psychiatry* 182: (Supplement 44).

Waldman. I.D. and Rhee, S.H. (2007) 'Genetic and Environmental Influences on Psychopathy and Anti-Social Behaviour'. In: C.J. Patrick (ed.), *Handbook of Psychopathy*. New York: Guilford Press. (Ch. 11).

Walker, N. (1968) *Crime and Insanity in England: The Historical Perspective*. (Vol. 1.) Edinburgh: University Press.

Walker, N. and McCabe, S. (1973) *Crime and Insanity in England: New Solutions and New Problems*. (Vol. 2.). Edinburgh: University Press.

Wambaugh, J. (1989) *The Blooding*. London: Bantam.

West, D.J. (1982) *Delinquency: Its Roots, Careers and Prospects*. London: Heinemann.

West, D.J. and Farrington, D.P. (1973) *Who Becomes Delinquent?* London: Heinemann.

(1977) *The Delinquent Way of Life: Third Report of the Cambridge Study in Delinquent Development*. London: Heinemann.

Whorton, J.C. (2010) *The Arsenic Century: How Victorian Britain Was Poisoned at Home, Work and Play*. Oxford: Oxford University Press.

Willmot P. and Gordon, N. (2011) *Working Positively with*

Personality Disorder in Secure Settings: A Practitioner's Perspective. Chichester: Wiley-Blackwell.

Wilson D. (2013), *Mary Ann Cotton: Britain's First Female Serial Killer*, Hook: Waterside Press.

Winnicott, D.W. (1949) 'Hate in the Counter-Transference'. In *International Journal of Psychoanalysis*, 30: 14-17.

Wootton, B. (1980) 'Psychiatry, Ethics and the Criminal Law'. In *British Journal of Psychiatry*, 136: 525-532.

World Health Organisation (WHO) (1992) *The ICD 10 Classification of Mental and Behavioural Disorders: Clinical Descriptions and Diagnostic Guidelines*. Geneva: WHO.

Chronological List of Key Statutes

Lunacy Act 1890

Mental Deficiency Act 1913

Mental Deficiency Act 1927

Mental Treatment Act, 1930

Criminal Justice Act 1948

Mental Health Act 1959

Criminal Justice Act 1967

Mental Health Act 1983

Mental Health (Patients in the Community) Act 1995

Crime (Sentences) Act 1997

Human Rights Act 1998

Criminal Justice and Court Services Act 2000

Criminal Justice Act 2003

Domestic Violence, Crime and Victims Act 2004

Mental Health Act 2007

Glossary

ADHD Attention deficit hyperactivity disorder: *Chapter 2.*

AMHP Approved mental health professional: see *Chapter 3.*

Asperger's syndrome (aka autism spectrum disorder (ASD)) Condition in which the individual concerned has difficulty relating to or empathising with other people, including when reading social or interpersonal situations: see *Chapter 3.*

Assessment A process within which a trained person applies incidents or factors against criteria, standards, norms, etc. in order to predict the likelihood of a given outcome, e.g. someone re-offending; whether there is a risk to the public (hence also the term 'prediction score').

Bonding A term used to signify the forging of close ties, dependence, affection, etc., e.g. as between a mother and child or with some other significant person in someone's life, lack of which may cause or lead to, e.g. emotional or personal difficulties.

Cerebral cortex Related to the brain system. Hence, e.g. terms such as 'cortical under arousal' — a defect or malfunction of that system: see *Chapter 2.*

CJS Criminal justice system. A reference to the entire system including, e.g. the police. prosecutors, courts, prisons and probation. For a general guide, see *The Criminal Justice System: An Introduction* (Gibson B and Cavdino P; 3rd edn. 2008), Hook: Waterside Press.

Crown Court The upper tier of trial courts in England and Wales that deals with the more serious criminal cases, i.e. above the level and jurisdiction of a magistrates' court. Only the Crown Court can restrict the discharge of mental health patients as described in *Chapters 3* and *4*.

Department of Health The Government Department with overall responsibility for public health, adult social services and the NHS and in a criminal justice context mental health services in relation to prisons and secure hospitals, as well as partnerships with other bodies working in similar fields: see generally www.dh.gov.ukPublic health, adult social care, and the NHS

DPD Dissocial personality disorder. One coming to attention due to a gross disparity between behaviour and social norms as outlined in *Chapter 2*.

DSPD Dangerous and severe personality disorder. A (non-medical) term used by Government in legislation (and now only historically there) to denote a particular degree or level of 'personality disorder' justifying certain state interventions: see *Chapters 1* and *2*.

DSM IV The *Diagnostic and Statistical Manual of Mental Disorders*: see *Chapter 2*.

ECT Electro-convulsive therapy: *Chapter 4*.

EEG Electro-encephalogram: *Chapter 2*.

GPI General paralysis of the insane: See *Chapter 2*.

Hare's Psychopathy Checklist: see *Psychopathy Checklist-Revised*

HMPS Her Majesty's Prison Service.

Home Office The Government Department with overall responsibility for criminal policy, the police and immigrations services (among other law and order related matters) and that until 2008 took responsibility for the mental health aspects of criminal justice alongside the *Department of Health*: see generally *The New Home Office: An Introduction* (2nd ed. 2008), Gibson B, Hook: Waterside Press and www.homeoffice.gov.uk

Hospital order A court order that an offender be admitted to hospital: see *Chapter 4.*

Huntingtons disorder (formerly 'chorea') An inherited terminal wasting disease of the mind: See *Chapter 2.*

ICD 10 *The International Classification of Mental and Behavioural Disorders*: see *Chapter 2.*

LHB Local Health Board: *Chapter 4.*

Limbic system Bodily system which is believed to be located in the upper brain stem and that controls brain processes—and which may be 'attacked', e.g. by infection: *Chapter 2.*

Metabolic Appertaining to the body itself, as e.g. when there are metabolic changes which affect behaviour: see *Chapter 2.*

MHA Mental Health Act (e.g. 1959; 1983; 2007): see *Chapters 2* and *3.*

MHRT Mental Health Review Tribunal: see *Chapters 3* and *4.*

MHS Mental health services. An informal term covering all types of provision.

MHT Mental health tribunal: see *Chapters 3 and 4.*

Ministry of Justice The Government Department (newly created in 2008) with responsibility for justice-related matters such as the running of the courts, prisons, human rights and related mental health services, the latter in conjunction with the *Department of Health* (above): see generally *The New Ministry of Justice: An Introduction* (2nd ed. 2008), Gibson B, Hook: Waterside Press and www. justice.gov.uk

MRI Magnetic resonance imaging, in the present context scanning the human brain to discern any disease that may lie within it; or possible unusual brain activity.

NPS National Probation Service (part of the National Offender Management Service (NOMS)). Any reference to the work of probation officers in this volume should be understood as being to their responsibilities under the general auspices of the NPS.

Neuro A term used to signify brain-related matters, as in 'neuro-physio-psychological' or 'neuroanatomy': see *Chapters 1* and *2*.

Parole Release on parole, as discussed in *Chapter 4*. Hence also **Parole Board**, **parole licence** (containing **parole conditions**), etc.

PCT Primary Care Trust.

PJ *Probation Journal: The Journal of Community and Criminal Justice.*

Prediction score See under *Assessment* above.

Presenting A term used to signify the symptoms or signs which a patient or subject displays (i.e. presents) to, e.g. a doctor, psychiatrist, psychologist or other person making an assessment (e.g. of level of risk).

PSJ *Prison Service Journal.* Nationwide magazine of *HMPS* (above).

Psychiatry A medical specialism concerned with the study, diagnosis, treatment and prevention of mental illnesses and disorders. Hence also 'psychiatrist'. The main distinction between a psychiatrist and a psychologist is that the former is qualified in medicine and is, e.g. empowered to prescribe or administer drugs as required, whereas a psychologist (see further below) is not.

Psychology An academic and practical discipline concerned with the scientific study of mental states, functions and related actions. Hence also 'psychologist'. A psychologist (of which there are many varieties) trains in psychiatry but compared to a psychiatrist is to an extent a 'lay' person, i.e. he or she is non-medically qualified. He or she will have a degree or degrees in psychology and will normally be involved in non-medical treatments (e.g. counselling in its various forms). Training as a clinical psychologist usually involves a higher degree such as a 'masters', or for certain types of clinical work (particularly in the forensic field) a doctorate (Ph.D).

Psychopathy A severe personality disorder variously characterised by a number of indicators, incidents or criteria such as those set out in the **Psychopathy Checklist-Revised** (Aka Hare's Psychopathy Checklist after Robert Hare: see *Chapters 4* and *5*): A frequently used forensic tool (there are others or variants) for assessing whether someone has a psychopathic personality—whether he or she has a 'score' (see below) high enough to require classification as a psychopath or further investigation and assessment of risk. The 20 criteria in Hare's checklist are (paraphrased/summarised):

- Glibness/superficial charm.
- Grandiose sense of self-worth.
- Proneness to boredom/Need for stimulation.
- Pathological lying.

- Conning/manipulative.
- Lack of remorse or guilt.
- Shallow affect.
- Callousnous/lack of empathy.
- Parasitic lifestyle.
- Poor behavioural controls.
- Promiscuous sexual behaviour.
- Early behaviour problems.
- Lack of realistic long term goals.
- Impulsivity.
- Irresponsibility.
- Failure to accept responsibility for own actions.
- Many short-term marital relationships.
- Juvenile delinquency.
- Revocation of conditional release.
- Criminal versatility.

The Hare Psychopathy Checklist is scored on a 40 point scale, where the item receives zero if it does not fit the particular criterion; one for a partial fit; and two if there is a reasonable fit. Normally only to be used by a trained professional, each item thus receives a score of 0-2 and the sum total of these scores is the critical indicator. The cut off for determination of a psychopathic personality is a score of 25 in Britain (30 in the USA).

RMO Responsible medical officer; although this term is no longer used by statute: see *Chapter 4*.

Restriction order The Crown Court (or an appellate court) may make an order restricting the discharge of an offender/patient from hospital where this is for the protection of the public from serious harm: see *Chapters 3* and *4*.

Secure provision A general term covering all levels of secure facilities for mentally disordered offenders or those unfit to stand trial: high security, semi-secure and low secure accommodation: *Chapter 4*.

Social services Ordinarily a reference to *local* social services, i.e. as provided by a local authority as opposed to central government or e.g. the *NPS* (above). The *Department of Health* (above) has certain related functions and responsibilities at national level.

SPD Severe personality disorder (whether or not *DSPD* above).

Special hospital This now redundant official description has been replaced by 'High security hospital', examples of which are Broadmoor and Rampton: *Chapter 4*.

Supervision Usually meaning supervision in the community under a court order or prison release license, parole licence or life licence (the later for life sentence prisoners): *Chapter 4*.

TC Therapeutic community: A grouping of people (large or small but in the present context in a hospital ward, a prison unit or wing, or as part of a community-based TC). Members of a TC discuss with and react to one another as a way of 'talking through' their situation with a view to resolving personal issues, such as those relating to addiction, anger, behaviour, (sometimes serious) offending or defects in personality— usually meaning under professional guidance and supervision.[1]

Toxic Poisonous, here meaning in relation to humans affected by a noxious substance, such as arsenic, mercury or lead in the

---

1. For in-depth accounts of 'whole' prison-based TCs in operation, see *Grendon Tales: Stories from a Therapeutic Community* (2001), Smartt, U and *Dovegate: A Therapeutic Community in a Private prison and Developments in Therapeutic Work with Personality Disordered Offenders* (2011), Cullen E and Mackenzie, J, both Hook: Waterside Press.

atmosphere or which has somehow entered the body, and which may affect the brain and behaviour: see *Chapter 2*.

Transfer The transfer from prison to hospital of prisoners found to be mentally disordered (and vice-versa although this is often described as 'being remitted' from hospital to prison): *Chapter 4*.

unit A general term used to describe a part or section of an organization, prison, hospital, facility, etc. that focuses on a given or 'dedicated' task, or on providing a particular service.

WHO World Health Organization. See www.who.int/en/

Index

> 'In a field prone to disappointment and disillusion he continues to stimulate and inspire': Sir Michael Day OBE
>
> 'I can think of no-one more instrumental at the pivotal meeting point of crime, criminal justice and mental disorder': Andrew Rutherford
>
> 'A monument to unassertive sanity': Sir Louis Blom-Cooper QC

Mad, Bad and Dangerous to Know
Reflections of a Forensic Practitioner
by Herschel Prins, Foreword by David Wilson

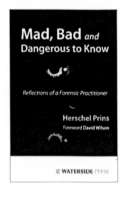

From a relatively modest background, Herschel Prins rose to become a leading authority on forensic work with offenders suffering from mental disorder.

In this frank and heartfelt account, he traces his journey from 'main grade' probation officer, Home Office civil servant, trainer and inspector to top level positions within academic institutions (notably at Leicester University and Loughborough University), with the Parole Board, key nationwide committees, inquiries and beyond.

'One of my heroes': Professor David Wilson

164 pages | Paperback & Ebook | Published 01/03/2012 | ISBN 978-1-904380-79-5

www.WatersidePress.co.uk/madbad